Praise for *Thanks for the Mammogram!*

"*Thanks for the Mammogram!* will give anyone going through breast cancer what they need most: courage, hope, and some much-needed laughs! By sharing her story, Laura Jensen Walker reminds all of us that while cancer is not funny, life often is, and sometimes laughter really is the best medicine!"

—OLYMPIC SKATER PEGGY FLEMING JENKINS, BREAST CANCER SURVIVOR

"Very informative, but also most definitely positive and uplifting for all women who have to face the terrible trials and tribulations of breast cancer. [The author's] genuine sense of humor shows how keeping a positive attitude is so important. I also really enjoyed the chapter penned by her husband. Certainly we husbands go through our own trauma with breast cancer when it affects our wives and those close to us."

—GREG JENKINS, M.D., HUSBAND OF PEGGY FLEMING

"I couldn't put this book down. A powerful demonstration of a patient's ability to defeat a disease we all hate. The author's approach needs to be deeply incorporated in treatment plans offered by conventional therapies. A must read for patients, physicians, and all those involved in the care of breast cancer—this book will bring peace to those so desperately in need of it."

—ERNIE BODAI, M.D., CREATOR OF THE BREAST CANCER AWARENESS POSTAGE STAMP

"One of the most powerful and effective tools in the cancer war chest is humor. And Laura Jensen Walker is masterful at wielding this painless and indispensable weapon in her wonderfully written book, *Thanks for the Mammogram!* She doesn't gloss over the weightier issues of the cancer battle, she simply brings balance to them through her use of humor and truths in God's Word."

—JAN DRAVECKY, VICE PRESIDENT, DAVE DRAVECKY'S OUTREACH OF HOPE, NATIONAL CANCER MINISTRY

"The best medicine for what ails us is often a hopeful, hilarious, compassionate survivor/companion to hold our hand through the dark valley. No one need walk through breast cancer alone. Laura is the perfect 'bosom buddy' for the journey—via the laughter, tears, and helpful information in *Thanks for the Mammogram!*"

—BECKY FREEMAN, NATIONAL SPEAKER AND AUTHOR OF *WORMS IN MY TEA*

"*Thanks for the Mammogram!* isn't for every woman. It's only for those who've experienced cancer, loved someone with cancer, met someone with cancer, worried about getting cancer, saw a made-for-TV movie about cancer once, read about cancer on a bus poster . . . in other words, honey, this book is for you. What an uplifting, uproarious approach to an otherwise serious, scary subject. Buy a copy for every woman you know!"

—LIZ CURTIS HIGGS, AUTHOR OF *HELP! I'M LAUGHING AND I CAN'T GET UP* AND *BAD GIRLS OF THE BIBLE*

"We don't always understand the twists and turns in our journey through this life, but in this book Laura Jensen Walker reminds us that faith in God and a good sense of humor help to keep us on the road and out of the ditch. If you or anyone you know is facing a challenge, this book is an epistle of encouragement . . . and a lot of laughs, too."

—MARTHA BOLTON, COMEDY WRITER AND AUTHOR OF *I LOVE YOU . . . STILL*

"Laura has pulled off an almost impossible feat—assaulting cancer with a massive dose of humor. And she won! This is an incredibly real, sensitive, gritty, hopeful book, woven through and through with Laura's signature brand of humor. It is far more than good entertainment—it is good medicine."

—DAVE MEURER, AUTHOR, *THE DAZE OF OUR WIVES: A SEMI-HELPFUL GUIDE TO MARITAL BLISS*

"I never thought of the word 'thanks' before in regard to my mammogram until Laura Jensen Walker readjusted my thinking. Now, I'm saying 'thanks' to Laura for reminding us how very funny life can be even in the midst of its most devastating interferences."

—SUE BUCHANAN, SPEAKER, AUTHOR OF *I'M ALIVE AND THE DOCTOR'S DEAD . . . SURVIVING CANCER WITH YOUR SENSE OF HUMOR AND YOUR SEXUALITY INTACT,* AND BREAST CANCER SURVIVOR

Thanks for the Mammogram!

Fighting Cancer with Faith, Hope, and a Healthy Dose of Laughter

Laura Jensen Walker

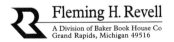
Fleming H. Revell

A Division of Baker Book House Co
Grand Rapids, Michigan 49516

Published by Fleming H. Revell
a division of Baker Book House Company
P.O. Box 6287, Grand Rapids, MI 49516-6287

Printed in the United States of America

Library of Congress Cataloging-in-Publication Data

Walker, Laura Jensen.
    Thanks for the mammogram! : fighting cancer with faith, hope, and a healthy dose of laughter / Laura Jensen Walker.
       p.   cm.
    ISBN 0-8007-1778-3 (cloth)
    1. Walker, Laura Jensen—Health. 2. Breast—Cancer—Patients—United States—Biography. I. Title.

RC280.B8 W33 2000
362.1'9699449—dc21
[B]   00-031081

For current information about all releases from Baker Book House, visit our web site:
                http://www.bakerbooks.com

For Mom, with love and gratitude

and in memory of Erma Bombeck
and of these who have gone on ahead . . .

Whatever is true,
Marita Brys
whatever is noble,
Lil Hooper
whatever is right,
Laura Kehoe
whatever is pure,
Stephanie Suzanne Sheely
whatever is lovely,
Kia Margaret Stirk
whatever is admirable—
Carla Anne Valles
if anything is excellent
Jane Valenzuela
or praiseworthy—
Pat Walter
think about such things.
—PHILIPPIANS 4:8

Contents

Contents

Foreword

When Laura Jensen Walker asked me to write an intro-
duction to this book, I felt honored. After all, I was Laura's
medical oncologist. I wrote the orders for the high dose
of chemotherapy Laura received as part of a National Cancer Institute sponsored clinical trial. I saw Laura in the
best and in the worst of times. I put her to the ultimate
test, and she still managed to crack a joke to cheer me up
and help others.

Thanks for the Mammogram! is the poignant, personal
account of Laura's encounter with breast cancer, and by
necessity, the medical establishment. Laura, the con-
summate journalist, questioned and probed, seeking
answers to the unknown. She never once wavered in her
determination to live and enjoy life to its fullest.

My first reading of the manuscript touched me deeply
as I relived some of the terrifying and even humorous
moments of Laura's battle against breast cancer. As Laura
states, "Cancer isn't funny," but she finds humor and
hope in everyday situations, touching the hearts of all
around her—friends, family, nurses, and yes, even doctors. During her darkest and scariest moments Laura

always managed a good word, a smile, a bit of hope. She never lost her faith.

To me, *Thanks for the Mammogram!* is not just a chronicle of cancer-related events—it is much more. It is about how Laura's family, friends, faith, and humor kept her together, whole, and sane during that awful period of "temporary insanity" we call adjuvant chemotherapy.

I know you will chuckle and cry, and cry and chuckle, when you read this book. And I can think of nothing more beautiful, for this is true life.

Vincent Caggiano, M.D.

Acknowledgments

This book was the hardest one I've written (of the legion of three I've penned so far) and the one closest to my heart. It could never have happened without the love and support of the following people.

First, to my husband and soulmate, Michael, you are the best gift God's ever given me. Thanks, honey, for reliving what was such a difficult time for you and then so eloquently and honestly transferring those memories to your own chapter, "Her Body, His Pain." We make a great team—on and off the page. Let's collaborate again, but next time not while under the pressure of three competing deadlines.

To my mom, Bettie Eichenberg, a fifteen-year breast cancer survivor who's always been my biggest cheerleader: Thank you for everything, including the welcome sustenance of those great homecooked meals during final deadline crunch. (Michael's stomach thanks you too.)

To my sister, Lisa: Thanks for all the last-minute medical expertise—and for spelling areola correctly.

Special thanks to the breast cancer survivors who so generously answered my questions and shared their cancer stories with me: Beverly Ann, Karen Chacon, Eve Dorf, Lynda Duncan, Bettie Eichenberg, Charlotte Frazier, Robyn Gibbons, Linda Gundy, Barbara Johnson, Nancy MaGuire, Barbara Nichols, Bonnie Sheaffer, Beverly Pierce Stroebel, "Aunt" Annette Sura, Debbie Thomas, Lee Tincher, Janis Whipple, and Sherris White. Thank you for your candor and your courage. This is your book too.

Eve, thanks also for sharing with me your beautiful artwork, which provided the inspiration for the title of this book.

Many thanks, as always, to Lana, who gives new meaning to the words *unconditional love.*

To the compassionate oncology nurses at Sutter Cancer Center and Mercy General Hospital of Sacramento—you guys are the best! Thank you for your tender care. (And Lisa, I still covet your thick, gorgeous waist-length hair. Wanna swap?)

Warm gratitude also goes to my skilled and caring doctors and surgeons: Vincent Caggiano, Virginia Hawes, Debra Johnson, and Karin Klove. Dr. Caggiano, you're a prince among oncologists.

To our retired medical friends, Chuck and Nela Hammel: Thank you for your availability and willingness to answer our oncology questions during the first frightening days after diagnosis. A special thanks for supporting Michael throughout that trying time.

Ditto to Sheri. We love you.

To Steve Laube who saw the need for this book and encouraged me to write it. Steve, live long and prosper.

To Susan Yates and Tom Thompson of Yates and Yates: Thank you for your unwavering belief in this project from the very beginning.

Deepest gratitude to my wonderful editor—and new friend—Lonnie Hull DuPont who caught the vision for this book, saw its potential, and buoyed me with her enthusiasm. Special thanks to Art Director Cheryl Van Andel and designer Gayle Raymer for the wonderful cover! To Lonnie, Cheryl, and the rest of the Revell team: Thank you for taking a chance and for making this dream a reality (with special thanks also to Twila Bennett, publicity wunderkind).

As always, my heartfelt thanks to Katie Young, my extraordinarily talented poet friend, who always acts as first reader on my books and continually pushes me to "be funny" even when I don't "feel" funny at the time. Katie, you deserve a medal for reading all those first drafts and for putting up with my (occasional) whining. Thanks too for my annual Sebastopol writing getaway and your to-die-for chocolate chip cookies.

Above all, thank you, God, for giving me life and guiding my pen.

Introduction

And if I laugh at any mortal thing,
  'Tis that I may not weep.

—Lord Byron

Cancer isn't funny.

But humor is healing.

As someone who has gone through breast cancer—mastectomy, chemotherapy, and reconstruction—and gratefully come out the other side, okay, a little lopsided, I've learned firsthand that laughter helps.

Big time.

From baldly going to where I'd never gone before to losing thirty pounds in thirty days the chemo diet way, humor has been an effective weapon in my fight against this disease that is no respecter of persons.

Almost everyone—whether it's your friend, neighbor, coworker, wife, mother, or sister—has been touched by breast cancer. The cancer survivors I've talked to over the years say that what helped them through their ordeal was faith and often humor.

I agree completely. But this is not to say that I laughed throughout my entire cancer experience.

I didn't.

There were days when I didn't find anything even remotely funny about it. (Think chemotherapy and emesis—barf—basin.) However, what helped me the most was when I could talk to other women who were going through the same thing. We'd compare mastectomy scars, swap funny wig stories, share how reconstruction affected our sex lives (saline implants have a tendency to pucker in certain, uh, situations), and simply laugh.

Yes, laugh.

There are those who are hesitant about the idea of cancer and humor. Some even think it's kind of "sick." But if you've been sick with cancer yourself or gone through it with a loved one, you know that laughter uplifts the soul.

And relieves tension.

It also lessens the fear and dread of those around you who don't know what to say or do. When I was going through cancer—more than eight years ago now, hurray!—I often found myself encouraging those who came to cheer *me* up. I'd put them at ease by joking about my flat chest or bald head: "I'm going for the less-is-more look these days."

Laughter helps.

So does talking to someone who's "been there."

Since my diagnosis, I've been asked by countless friends, relatives, friends of friends, and acquaintances to talk to a friend or loved one who's just discovered she has breast cancer. I'm always happy to, because someone did the same thing for me and it made all the difference.

This book, the one so near and dear to my heart, is an outgrowth of my desire to share my story and bits and pieces of other women's stories in hopes that they will help others.

I pray this book will convince women going through breast cancer—and those who love them—that faith, hope, and a healthy dose of laughter can make all the difference. Or at least provide some much-needed comic relief every now and then.

I also hope it will inspire women everywhere to get a mammogram today!

Daytime TV talk show host and "Queen of Nice" Rosie O'Donnell and I share that same mission. Rosie, whose mom died from breast cancer when she was young, does everything she can to demystify the fear of mammograms and increase breast cancer awareness.

Rosie and I share something else too: a love of Broadway show tunes and a penchant for making up songs. That woman will sing anytime, anyplace, about anything.

Sing out, Rosie, sing out!

Each October—Breast Cancer Awareness Month—she makes up and sings funny little ditties about mammograms on her show.

Well, I don't have a TV show, but I've made up a little mammogram song myself. C'mon now, everyone, sing out with me:

Thanks for the Mammogram
(sung to the tune of "Thanks for the Memories")

Thanks for the mammogram.
Though it hurt a little bit,
Okay, kind of a lot,
It's wonderful what it can do,
It found my cancer spot,
Now I'm cancer-free.
Thanks for the mammogram.
A small squish goes a long way
To finding the Big C.
It really can help save the life
Of folks like you and me.
Get your mam-mogram!

one

For Better or Worse

Bad news on our first wedding anniversary that was not part of our happily-ever-after plan.

Love is as strong as death, . . .
It burns like blazing fire,
like a mighty flame.
Many waters cannot quench love;
rivers cannot wash it away.
—SONG OF SONGS 8:6–7

On August 4, 1992, my husband, Michael, and I celebrated our first wedding anniversary.

Some couples get monogrammed stationery or season tickets to the ballet for that first (paper or plastic) anniversary; others get beautiful coffee-table books or colorful picnic ware.

I got cancer.

Not exactly a gift that can be returned.

It was the day after our anniversary when the doctor gave me the news.

CANCER was all I heard, and all I could think of was death. I was only thirty-five years old; I had finally graduated from college—and passed math—and was blissfully married to the man I'd been waiting for all my life.

How could this all be taken away?

It wasn't.

The only things taken away were a breast, some lymph nodes, the contents of my stomach, some weight I'd been trying to lose for years, and later, temporarily, my hair.

I felt the lump one warm summer night as Michael and I were lying in bed reading. As I reached up to push my hair out of my face, my hand inadvertently brushed against my breast, and I felt something hard.

"Honey, I just felt something strange," I said absently, using my fingers to try to locate the firm little knot I'd grazed while still keeping my eyes glued to my Agatha Christie novel.

"Maybe it's a tumor," I teased, quoting a line from the Arnold Schwarzenegger comedy, *Kindergarten Cop.*

"It's not a too-mah," Michael joked back in his best Arnold imitation.

Suddenly, I found it—a hard, round lump about the size of a pea. My reading stopped abruptly.

"Honey, I feel a lump," I said nervously.

"It's just your fiber-whatchamacallit," he reassured me. But then he leaned over to feel it too. We had a difficult time finding it again, however, since I have "lumpy" fibro-cystic breasts. We kept feeling the wrong lumps.

I relaxed, because if we had a hard time telling one lump from another, then it was probably nothing. But a few seconds later we finally located it. Michael agreed that this lump did feel a bit different.

The next morning, I called my doctor for an appointment and went to see her a couple days later.

She couldn't find the lump at first either. But once she did, she told me it was probably just a water-filled cyst or a side effect of too much caffeine. She told me to cut down my caffeine intake and scheduled a mammogram "just to be on the safe side."

Now I've never been a coffee drinker, but touch my Earl Grey, and you're in hot water. So the idea of giving up my favorite "cuppa" tea with milk and sugar was more disturbing than the thought of the mammogram.

After all, what's a little breast-flattening and scrunching? It's not like I had much to scrunch.

Besides, I'd already had my first mammogram just a couple years earlier, when I was thirty-three, much to the surprise of the lab technicians who thought I was a bit young for one. However, due to my fibrocystic breasts and family history of breast cancer (my mom is a breast cancer survivor), I felt it was important.

That mammogram came back fine, and the lab techs assured me I was too young to worry about breast cancer, so I didn't need another mammogram for four or five years. Their medically learned advice, coupled with my tight budget, prohibited me from going back for a second one the following year.

I'm forever grateful I had that first baseline mammogram though. Now the lab had something to compare this one against, and there was a definite difference. That difference prompted the doctor to order a biopsy, again "just to be safe." She referred us to a wonderful surgeon, Dr.

Karin Klove, and we scheduled the biopsy for the following week—the day after our wedding anniversary.

The night of our anniversary Michael took me out for a lovely, romantic dinner, and we joyfully celebrated our first year together as husband and wife.

The next morning, Michael and my mom accompanied me to the surgery center for a routine biopsy.

As I came out of the anesthesia, Mom and Michael gripped my hands as Dr. Klove approached, but in my groggy state, that didn't even register. I smiled and nodded drowsily as she explained her findings. It wasn't until she gently said, "I'm afraid it's cancerous," that the grogginess disappeared—in a skipped heartbeat.

CANCER?

Cancer *kills* people! I didn't want to die, not now. It was too soon. I was too young. And I was still a newlywed.

Tears of terror fell from my eyes as Michael and my mom tightened their grip on my hands reassuringly.

Dr. Klove told me she was encouraged by the small size of the lump—1.5 centimeters—because that meant it was caught early. She talked to us for a few more minutes, mentioning different options and suggesting we stop by her office in a couple days to pick up some educational breast cancer literature.

Meanwhile, Michael excused himself to call his sister who was waiting for news. (It wasn't until much later that

I learned he completely fell apart on the phone.) When he returned, my tears were gone, and so were his, and the journalist in me had taken over. "Okay, let's go get all that information now so we can research and study what to do next," I said practically.

Looking back, I see God's grace in that moment.

Practicality has never been my strong suit—I've been called the world's biggest dreamer—so even though I had a degree in journalism, I preferred writing "people" or feature stories, rather than hard news. And even though I loved *All the President's Men* and briefly dreamed of being the next Woodward or Bernstein, Erma Bombeck was my real hero.

But in that moment, God used my journalism training to get my focus off my fears.

After I dressed, Michael and I drove straight to Dr. Klove's office to pick up the information, which we pored over and prayed over that night.

We briefly discussed a lumpectomy, but I'd heard stories of women who had gone the lumpectomy route only to have more cancer discovered in the same breast later. Then they still needed a mastectomy. I decided to cut right to the chase and go the modified radical mastectomy route.

In recent years, many research studies have shown that lumpectomies followed by radiation have the same effectiveness as mastectomies, and I know women who've had them and are doing great. But were I to be diagnosed with breast cancer today, I'd probably still opt for a mastectomy.

It's a personal choice. But for me and my peace of mind, it was the right decision, especially because I had a very aggressive type of cancer.

I don't see mastectomy as mutilation; I see it as necessary. If I had gangrene in my leg, surgeons would cut off the leg to save my life. That was the same way I viewed a mastectomy.

My life is much more important to me than my breast.

Michael lovingly assured me that whatever choice I made, he would support me completely. He never pushed one way or another. He just made it abundantly clear that he wanted me around for many years; whatever it took to ensure that was fine with him.

Besides, he hadn't married me for my breasts. He'd married me for my artistic nature, my sense of humor, and my ability to beat him at Silver Screen Trivial Pursuit.

The night before my mastectomy, we went out to dinner with my entire family. Everyone was concerned and serious.

Too serious for me.

At one point, my teenage nephew Josh dropped his steak knife, so I gave him mine. He cut a big bite of steak, and the fork was halfway to his mouth when I said, "Oops. Hope you don't catch cancer from using my knife."

That lightened the mood considerably. Although I can't say what it did for Josh's appetite.

Humor helps.

Later that night, as Michael and I were lying in bed, I looked down at my breasts. Suddenly something came over me.

A song (sung to the tune of "Bye, Bye, Birdie").

> *Bye, bye, boo-by . . . I hate to see you go.*
> *Bye, bye, booby. It won't be much of a blow.*

Michael joined in on the second verse:

> *No more boo-by, we're sad to see you go.*
> *Bye, bye, boo-by, let's get on with the show.*

Show tunes were one of the things that first drew Michael and me together, and they didn't fail us now.

The following year on our anniversary, I fractured my elbow.

It was two years before we celebrated another anniversary.

> *A cheerful heart is good medicine,*
> *but a crushed spirit dries up the bones.*
> —Proverbs 17:22

two

Beauty and the Breast

Also known as reconstruction or the "build-a-breast" route. Kind of like Lego's™, except the pieces don't snap together.

How poor are they that have not patience!
What wound did ever heal but by degrees?

—WILLIAM SHAKESPEARE

In the aftermath of the Civil War, the fallen South underwent a period known as Reconstruction, as the government reorganized the Confederate states that had seceded from the Union.

In the aftermath of my initial skirmish with cancer, I also underwent a period of reconstruction. Prior to mastectomy, I had to decide whether I wanted reconstructive surgery, or the "build-a-breast" route as Michael and I called it. Kind of like Lego's™, except the pieces didn't snap together.

A boob job? Me? Never in a million years.

After all, plastic surgery was for models and actresses who made their living with their looks. And I'd always made mine with my mind—and my big mouth.

Besides, this whole reconstruction process seemed like a long, drawn-out affair to me, and I really didn't want any more pain than was necessary. Or to have my cancer experience last even one minute longer than required.

So I was tempted to say, "Forget it. Just cut off my breast and be done with it."

But then a friend who had undergone a double mastectomy followed by reconstruction dropped by to visit me.

This friend is in her mid-thirties, petite, small-boned, and very attractive. You'd never know from looking at her that she'd had her breasts replaced. But just so I could have an idea of how a rebuilt breast looked, she opened her blouse for me.

I still didn't notice anything different—except that she didn't have my love handles. She was wearing a beautiful black lacy bra and looked like a model for a Victoria's Secret ad.

Then she undid her bra.

Wow.

Talk about the miracles of modern medicine. She looked great. And so did they.

I was really impressed. She confided that she especially liked her new set because her old pair had begun to feel the pull of gravity. But even though her breasts looked terrific, I still didn't want to base my decision purely on a visual thing.

My mom was the turning point.

About a decade earlier, when Mom was in her early fifties, she'd undergone two mastectomies within two years. She said that if her insurance had covered it and she'd been a little younger, she definitely would have chosen reconstructive surgery. Without it, every morning and night when she dresses and undresses, she's faced with a daily reminder of the disease.

That clinched it.

I didn't want cancer to have its control over me any longer than was absolutely necessary. I wanted to take the steps I needed to get rid of it and continue on with my life.

I decided to meet with a plastic surgeon.

As Michael and I walked into the plush waiting room of the plastic surgery center, all I saw were thin, gorgeous bodies and smooth, shiny faces. I felt a bit out of place with my crow's feet and thunder thighs until I noticed a couple regular-looking women wearing hats or wigs. "Comrades!" I longed to shout.

Once inside the examination room, the nurse had me remove everything from the waist up. She handed me a beautiful silky print kimono to put on—a vast improvement over those paper-flat blue "gowns" that are always such a pain to open, often ripping in the process.

So *that's* where all the money from those nose jobs goes.

The nurse left while I changed and returned a few minutes later with a camera. I had to open that pretty robe and reveal my no-longer-youthful bosoms so she could snap a picture.

Talk about a Kodak moment.

Shortly afterward, the plastic surgeon, a vivacious, attractive woman about my age, examined me. When we rejoined Michael in her office, she explained the different options available.

"Are you considering a prophylactic mastectomy?" she asked.

Prophylactic? I thought that was for preventing pregnancy or disease.

Turns out prophylactic *is* for prevention—the prevention of cancer in the remaining healthy breast. She said that some women were choosing to have their "good" breast removed at the same time as the "bad" one so they wouldn't have to worry about getting cancer in the second breast later.

"You mean get rid of the other one too even though there's nothing wrong with it?" I asked. That seemed just a little too radical to me. I mean, why fix it if it's not broken?

I decided to pass on the prophylactic.

Next, she pulled out this pinkish mound thing with a Jell-O-like consistency that looked remarkably like a breast and handed it to Michael to feel. It was hard to tell which was pinker: the silicone implant or Michael's face.

But he bravely assumed his most clinical air and scientifically examined the implant before quickly passing it over to me.

Although the silicone implant felt remarkably like a real breast, I decided to go with a saline implant instead. Even though it didn't look and feel as real as silicone, I figured a little salt water couldn't hurt if the implant ever ruptured or was accidentally punctured.

My reconstruction began in the operating room at the same time as the mastectomy. Immediately after my breast was removed, my plastic surgeon, Dr. Debra Johnson, inserted a tissue expander into my chest to stretch the tissue to make room for the saline implant that would later be inserted. After recuperating from surgery, I would go in on a regular basis for "fill-ups."

The tissue expander starts out like a flat balloon.

At my weekly expansions, Dr. Johnson would take a tiny magnet attached to a string and circle my wannabe breast until she found the exact location of the metallic entry point on the tissue expander beneath my muscle.

I was always tempted to say, "Contact. Start your syringes."

Once she made contact, she'd fill an enormous syringe with saline and "pump me up."

I'd been told there'd be "some discomfort" as the tissue expanded, but no one said it would feel like I had a Frisbee™ jammed inside my chest.

Also, it takes a while for everything to "settle" into place, so until it did, I looked like the hunchbreast of Notre Dame.

Good thing Michael's got a sense of humor.

And can sing.

I love Michael's voice. In fact, the first time I ever saw him he was singing a song that made me cry. The words touched my heart, but it was his interpretation of the music that really moved me. My actor-husband puts a lot of passion into his singing, and it shows.

Since we've been married, he's serenaded me on several occasions much to my delight.

One night during the beginning stages of my bosom remodeling we'd been acting silly and goofing around when he looked over at me with an impish grin and soulfully began to sing (to the tune "Memory" from *CATS*):

> *Mammary, all alone in the moonlight,*
> *I can dream of the old days;*
> *there were two of you then.*
> *I remember . . . a time I knew what happiness was;*
> *let the mammary live again.*

I laughed until I cried.

Don't you just love a man who can belt out a Broadway show tune?

The most fascinating part of my breast remodeling/reconstruction was the creation of my new nipple.

Dr. Johnson made a crosslike incision in the center of my tissue-expanded hump, folded the edges to the center, and stitched around the base of the circle so that a slight protuberance formed. Previously, she'd tattooed the "Oreo" (areola) area to make it look more lifelike. She told me she'd had to visit tattoo parlors as part of her training to learn the technique.

When my friends learned about my tattoo, they started calling me "Lydia, Lydia, the tattooed lady."

Different doctors use different construction methods.

Some remove and save the original nipple and sew it to the woman's side, which made me wonder if they were afraid of losing it or something. But I could just imagine

Michael waking up in the middle of the night and seeing this Cyclops winking at him. I later learned that, with this method, doctors grafted the nipple onto the skin so it would continue to receive the necessary nutrition from the blood to remain healthy.

Tattooing seemed a tad tamer to me.

About a year after my reconstruction was complete, I was matron-of-honor in my best friend's wedding. I was thrilled to be able to stand up for her, but I was almost equally as thrilled by my dress—a pretty, off-the-shoulder, slightly low-cut navy and white lace number.

"Look," I boasted to friends as I proudly leaned over their table at the reception—"cleavage!"

She is clothed with strength and dignity;
she can laugh at the days to come.
—Proverbs 31:25

three

To Baldly Go Where I'd Never Gone Before

Bald is beautiful. If Capt. Jean-Luc Picard, Michael Jordan, and Yul Brynner can look good bald, why can't I?

Humor is a prelude to faith and
Laughter is the beginning of prayer.
—REINHOLD NIEBUHR

Yul Brynner, Michael Jordan, Capt. Jean-Luc Picard—all baldly went where "no one had gone before."

Why couldn't I?

Just because I'm a woman, who says I need hair to look good? After all, week after week on *Star Trek: The Next Generation*, women swooned in front of their TVs over the tea-drinking, Shakespeare-quoting, BALDING Patrick Stewart as Captain Picard. He even made the cover of *TV Guide* as "Sexiest Man on TV."

At least my chrome dome and I would be in good company.

Besides, after going through the debilitating days of chemo, becoming bald was a breeze.

At first, I didn't think I'd lose my hair, because the doctor said that usually happened eight to ten days after chemotherapy. And by day nine, all my hair was still firmly in place. On the tenth day, however, as I bent over to unload the dishwasher, my head suddenly began to itch. I reached up to scratch it, and a fine shower of brown hair rained down on the stark white open dishwasher door.

Yuck!

A rather disgusting sight for a fastidious woman who can't stand to see even one hair in the bathroom sink.

Something my eagle eye always zeroes in on whenever Michael finishes trimming his beard. Yes, he cleans up after himself, but somehow, three or four whiskers always manage to elude him.

He says I'm splitting hairs.

Once I realized I was losing my hair, I made an appointment with the barber down the street to shave it off.

One of the worst things about cancer is the control it has over your body. You feel powerless. Although I know that God is in control of every facet of my life, I was used to commanding my body to do what I wanted.

But cancer robs you of that illusion.

Additionally, my oncologist had said that those people who had a defeatist attitude and just let cancer have its way didn't fare as well as those patients who, even in the tiniest way, exerted some control over the disease.

Deciding to get my head buzzed instead of waiting until all my hair fell out was my way of exerting a modicum of control. Unfortunately, when I called the barber after my dishwasher downpour, I learned he wouldn't be able to fit me in until the next day.

By now my head was itching like crazy.

Not my whole head though, just pockets.

I'd reach up to scratch and come away with clumps of hair in my hand. After a couple hours, it became second nature to scratch, get a clump, and throw it away, scratch-get-a-clump-throw-it-away.

That night, our friends Dave and Pat Smith, who were visiting from England, dropped by for a casual get-together.

They were joined by our mutual friends Pat and Ken McLatchey. Ken, or Captain McLatchey as I used to call him, was my former boss when we were both stationed with the Air Force in England.

We were all having a great time, laughing and reminiscing about our days in "Merrie Olde," when I began to absentmindedly scratch my head to relieve the insatiable itching. Naturally, a clump of hair came away in my hand; without thinking, I slipped into automatic pilot and repeated the scratch-get-a-clump-throw-it-away routine I'd been practicing all day.

Only now I didn't have a place to throw away the hair without being rude and getting up every few seconds to go to the bathroom.

Instead, I oh-so-casually yet surreptitiously stretched my arm out along the back of the couch and began dropping handfuls of hair behind it. I didn't want to interrupt the flow of conversation, and besides, I figured no one would notice. Later, after everyone left, I'd just sweep it up with no one the wiser.

Right.

All talk abruptly ceased as Ken suddenly said, "Laura, what ARE you doing?" Michael chimed in: "And she gets mad at *me* for leaving a couple hairs in the bathroom sink?"

Not one of my more shining moments. My only excuse was that we were in the privacy of our home with friends with whom I felt very comfortable, so I scratched without thinking.

The chemo made me do it.

Really.

I have it on good authority—my girlfriends—that in addition to frying hair cells, the toxic chemicals in chemotherapy can fry brain cells.

Especially the ones that control etiquette.

It's not that my mother didn't raise me properly. She always said it was rude to interrupt when others are talking. Guess she just forgot to teach me that Emily Post part about pulling out my hair in front of company.

Not to worry though. The hair shedding would soon be a thing of the past.

When I called the barber to make an appointment for my buzz cut, I told him the reason for shaving my head was due to the side effects of chemotherapy, *not* because I was longing to be the next Sinead O'Connor. Deliberately choosing to hasten the balding process was difficult enough without having to deal with a lot of questions once I arrived at the shop.

Besides, a barbershop was not my normal turf; I usually had my hair cut and styled at a beauty salon. Yet every time I walked by the windows of this neighborhood barber, it looked empty, so I figured it would be a pretty painless and anonymous way to fulfill my mission.

Barbers are a lot cheaper too, and we were pinching our pennies in those days.

I didn't want Michael to go with me, because I didn't want his first sight of my hairless head to be in public. I preferred the privacy of our home for that.

I did take my mom along for moral support.

When we arrived at the barbershop, much to my dismay, three of the four chairs were occupied. And it was a different barber than the one I'd talked to the day before. He kept asking me, "Are you sure you want to do this? How about just a nice, short cut instead?"

Trying not to cry, I said quietly, "It's not a question of want, it's a question of need."

Finally, he started shaving my head. I kept my eyes lowered the entire time because I didn't want the first glimpse of my shorn scalp to be in a barbershop full of men.

When he was finished, my mom gently stroked my head and said admiringly, "You have a beautiful head—perfectly shaped with no dents or dings." But I couldn't bear to look at it just then, so I jammed on my corduroy hat, paid the barber, and left.

When we got home, Michael hurried in from the back room and asked gently, "How's it look?"

"I don't know," I said, nervously heading for the bathroom. As I pulled off my hat and looked into the mirror for the first time, I burst into tears at the Uncle Fester (*Addams Family*) face I didn't recognize.

"I look like a freak," I sobbed.

"No, you don't," my husband and my mom chorused.

Michael tenderly put his arm around me, meeting my tear-filled eyes in the mirror with eyes filled with love. "You're beautiful," he said softly. That's when my mom, a very perceptive woman, picked up her purse and discreetly left.

After the initial shock, I got used to my new "do" pretty quickly. The only problem was, I kept giving Michael whisker burns.

On the up side, I didn't have to spend any time in the morning blow drying or curling my hair. I just showered, used a dab of shampoo, rinsed, and dried. It was kind of fun rubbing my palm against my bristle-buzz. It was even better when all the tiny bristles finally fell out, and the surface was smooth to the touch.

Eventually, I lost every single hair on my body, including my eyebrows and eyelashes. One day as Michael and I passed the bathroom mirror clad only in our birthday suits, I was struck by the contrast and said, "Oh, look. It's cueball and furball."

Many women who lose their hair to chemotherapy choose the wig route.

I could have gotten a free wig through the American Cancer Society to cover my soon-to-be-Kojak coif, but every wig I tried on made me look like the Texas cheer-leader's mom. Since I've never been one for big hair, I opted for the Sigourney Weaver *Alien 3* look instead.

And I'm glad I did.

My Sigourney selection turned out to be a good choice. Dr. Caggiano, my oncologist, a sweet, kindly man in his sixties, upon seeing my shiny scalp for the first time and noticing the resemblance to the movie star, said: "I think she is one of the most beautiful women in Hollywood."

That man is really a gifted doctor.

The nurses were great too. They kept telling me I had a beautifully shaped head—no dents or dings. Recalling my mother saying almost exactly the same thing in the barbershop, I realized she must have coughed up big bucks to those oncology nurses.

One friend of mine, a little more on the cutting edge than most in our circle of friends, even told me I should keep my "hair" that way because it looked so good. Now I've been known to do some off-the-wall things in my time, but that sure wasn't going to be one of them.

The only problem with being bald is your head gets really cold.

To help out, friends and family kept buying or making me great hats and scarves.

My mom took me shopping and treated me to a trea-sure chest of beautiful silk scarves. My talented friend Susan made me a rich burgundy-print corduroy cloche and a pale-blue moire hat with ribbons and flowers. And Katie, my starving poet friend, splurged on an elegant, floppy, black velvet hat.

It became a fun game of dress up, just like when I was a little girl. One day I was a gypsy with a brightly colored scarf and flashing gold earrings; the next, I was Audrey Hepburn in a wide-brimmed straw hat.

One October morning when my day's ensemble was topped by a borrowed black felt bowler, I stopped to buy gas. When I went in to pay the convenience store clerk, she laughed and said, "What are *you* supposed to be?"

A bit taken aback until I realized it was Halloween, I smiled and said, "Liza Minnelli in *Cabaret*."

Laughter CAN be the best medicine.

And humor has always been an integral part of who I am; since God made me, I know that sense of humor comes from him. Why not make good use of what he has given?

God has also given us awareness. Statistics say that one in every eight women will get breast cancer sometime in their lives. Yes, that's frightening. But it's a fact. Hiding from it won't change it. What's even more frightening to me is fear.

Fear that prevents a woman from getting a lump checked when she first discovers it.

Fear that she'll be less of a woman without a breast.

Fear of the side effects of chemotherapy.

Fear that she'll be unattractive without hair.

One woman even told me that she'd be absolutely "humiliated" without her hair and would just stay inside her house throughout the whole ordeal if she went bald.

Not me.

I believe in confronting things head-on—pun intended. Granted, it took a bit of time getting used to my naked noggin, but once I did, I decided I might as well get a few laughs out of it. So whenever my head got too hot under my hat at work or in public, I'd just doff my cap and ask friends and coworkers if they wanted to feel my shiny dome.

Besides, the way I always looked at it, hair grows back. Your life doesn't.

The greater part of our happiness or misery depends on our dispositions and not on our circumstances.

—Martha Washington

four

How to Lose Thirty Pounds in Thirty Days: The Chemo Diet Way

The original Slim-Fast liquid diet.
(But not one I'd recommend.)

Always laugh when you can. It is cheap medicine.
—LORD BYRON

I've struggled with my weight since I was a teenager. The night before my Air Force pre-enlistment physical when I was nineteen, I popped a drugstore diet pill, wrapped my naked, quarter-pounder body in plastic kitchen wrap, and gingerly lowered myself into a tub of nearly scalding water in a last-ditch attempt to steam off two more pounds.

I really wanted Uncle Sam to want *me*.

And he did. He really did. I got in—and celebrated afterwards with a Snickers bar.

But three years later I found myself on the Air Force "fat girl" program. I've forgotten the real title, something very correct and official sounding, but all the GIs called it the fat-girl or fat-boy program.

One pound overweight could earn you a place in the program.

And I qualified. Uncle Sam didn't take kindly to overweight, unfit personnel. Guess it didn't fit into that lean-mean military machine image.

Since black-and-white penitentiary wear wasn't exactly my style (yes, being habitually "fat" was a court-martial offense), I became the diet queen. More than twenty years later, I still recall the aftereffects of those awful canned spinach-and-eggs lunches. I even—and this will surprise anyone who knows couch-potato me—began running three miles a day on my lunch hour.

Sometimes, all this effort just wasn't quite enough, however.

So I'd pop another diuretic the night before weigh-in. And just in case, I had one final trick under my uniform. My bra.

Since Uncle Sam subtracted three pounds for clothes, I'd always slip into the rest room first, remove my bra, and stuff it into my black, GI-issue purse before stepping on the scale.

Those were the times I longed for Dolly Parton's cups.

Her bra probably weighed a good five pounds. Easily.

Whereas mine generally managed to shave off just another three ounces.

If only I'd known about the "chemo diet" then. I could've lost thirty pounds in thirty days on the original slim-fast liquid diet. Although it's not a weight loss program I'd recommend.

Years later, when I found out I had cancer and would need chemotherapy, I opted to be part of a nationwide research study through the National Cancer Institute that was studying whether stronger chemotherapy in a shorter period of time was more effective. Rather than the normal six months to a year's worth of treatments, they scheduled four treatments over a three-month span.

As part of the study, the computer randomly selected which women would receive which dosage of chemo-therapy. The options were standard dosage, a combination of standard and heavy, and heavy heavy.

Well, the computer "randomly" selected me to get the "heavy heavy" dosage.

Only we know that God's not random. We believe I got the dose he knew I needed.

Dr. Caggiano told us that everyone responded differently to chemo, so there was no way to predict how I'd react.

On the upside, however, one of his patients, who preferred to remain private about her cancer and chemo-therapy treatments, did so well during chemo that her employer never even knew about it. She'd have her treatment late Friday, feel "flu-like" over the weekend, and return to work Monday with no one having a clue.

I'd heard of many other women who likened chemo to the flu—including noted journalist Linda Ellerbee. In a *TV Guide* article discussing her breast cancer and subsequent chemotherapy treatments a few years ago, she said chemo was like "working when you had the flu."

Not like any flu I've ever known.

I'd never retched every couple hours for eight days straight with the flu. The dictionary definition of *flu* is: "an acute, infectious viral disease characterized by inflammation of the respiratory tract, fever, muscular pain, and intestinal irritation."

Irritation?

My intestines weren't irritated, they were furious! This was war, and my stomach was the battlefield. Even a drink of water would send it into spasms.

I had to be hospitalized for each chemo stay because the dosage prescribed for me was so high. In fact, the night of the first treatment when the nurse read my chart, she thought there was some mistake. "This can't be right," she said. "I've never given a patient this high a dose before."

She called the doctor to check.

It was no mistake.

The mistake was made a few minutes later.

One of the other oncology nurses was supposed to give me Zofran, a relatively new "miracle" antinausea medication, *before* the chemo so it would have a chance to get in my body to counteract the toxic aftereffects of chemo that were known to wreak nausea havoc with the system.

Unfortunately, she misunderstood that the Zofran should have been administered first. By the time she realized her mistake, it was too late. The chemo had already entered my bloodstream. So, this wonderful "miracle drug" that relieved nausea in many cancer patients didn't do zip for me.

The morning after that first dose, I was not feeling too bad—a couple of baby twinges of nausea and that was it. My sister and nephew had stopped by to visit, and Michael was also in the room. I went into the bathroom, and while I was indisposed, it happened.

People always talk about "waves" of nausea. Well, if this was a wave, it would have to be put in the tidal wave class. Remember *The Poseidon Adventure*? It welled up from somewhere deep inside of me. And not only did it feel awful; it sounded awful.

Think *Jurassic Park* and the roar of the T-Rex.

In a flash, Michael was by my side with a basin and a cool cloth for my neck.

Now, I try to maintain my sense of humor at all times, but I must confess that I lost it—along with everything else inside me—during the chemo days.

During my second treatment I retched so forcefully that I broke blood vessels in my eyes, which I didn't even realize until I looked in the mirror.

Staring back at me was this pale, hairless, bloody-eyed, lopsided creature from the Black Lagoon whom I didn't recognize.

Can you say attractive?

Actually, the second treatment was probably the worst. In addition to bursting blood vessels, I had to have my IV removed and changed three times, with the lovely experience of being poked with a needle each time, because all the veins in my arm were collapsing.

That's when the medical staff decided to insert a PICC line (catheter)—a long flexible tubing the thickness of a swizzle stick—that they threaded up inside the veins of my arm to a larger vein inside my chest. The nurses gave me Novocain so I didn't feel a thing during the intricate procedure, but I couldn't bear to watch. So Michael, after sterilizing his hands and donning scrubs and a mask, did so, in clinical fascination.

"Wow, that is so cool," he said enthusiastically.

Ever notice that guys have a rapt interest in squeamish things?

The PICC line was a godsend, however. Now I had two painless entry ports sticking out of my arm—one where the nurses administered the chemo, the other where they drew my blood without having to stick me anymore.

That, I liked.

The constant throwing up, I didn't.

But I was an anomaly. My oncologist said that in all his years of practice, he'd never seen anyone affected as horribly by the chemo as I was. Nor had any of his colleagues at the cancer center.

I always knew I was unique.

After that second treatment when I continued to throw up for such a long period, my doctor recommended home health care and constant hydration after each hospitalization. A home health nurse came out to our house and hooked me up to a portable IV—using my brand-new

PICC line ports—which continued to give me fluids as well as antinausea medication.

It helped—some.

Now instead of throwing up every few hours for eight or nine days in a row, I only threw up every few hours for *six* days in a row.

The nurse showed Michael how to change my IV bags of saline and how to administer the antinausea medication. The latter came in a lightweight clear plastic oval the size of a baseball with the medication concentrated in a piece of surgical tubing in the center inflated like a water balloon. As the medication dispersed into my system, the water-balloon tubing deflated into a straight line.

Michael, my creative and utilitarian husband, saved the empty "chemo balls" because he thought they'd make great Christmas ornaments.

I told him he was a sick puppy.

My chemo experience wasn't all bad.

I did lose weight—a lot. Thirty pounds in thirty days.

For the first time in my life, I looked forward to stepping on the scale.

Michael noticed the change too. One night at home—in between chemo treatments—we were snuggling, when all of a sudden he felt something unusual. "What's that?" he asked, with a trace of fear in his voice.

"My hip bone!" I sang out joyfully.

Just call me Cindy Crawford.

I finished my last chemo treatment a couple weeks before Christmas. And Michael, that sentimental guy of mine who likes to remember the important moments in life, did something really special for Christmas.

He made me a chemo ball Christmas ornament complete with ribbons and pearls.

He will yet fill your mouth with laughter
and your lips with shouts of joy.
—JOB 8:21

five

Of Ice Chips, Suppositories, and Hospital "Hats"

The insurmountable joys of hospital life.

63

To me, every hour of the day and night is an unspeakably perfect miracle.

—Walt Whitman

Bonnie Sheaffer got the surprise of her life when she went in for her first radiation treatment.

Men without pants.

"The men who were undergoing treatment for prostate cancer had these little gowns on instead of their pants, and they were in the same room with women—like me—who had only one breast and were wearing *their* little gowns," Bonnie recalled.

"At first I thought 'oh, my goodness,' but then I got used to it and wound up becoming the informal social director, introducing all the new people that came in," she said.

You get used to lots of what-were-once-embarrassing things when you're being treated for cancer.

Like throwing up.

Suppositories.

And hospital "hats."

Now I got a lot of pretty hats when I was going through chemo, but this hospital number was in a class all its own.

White and plastic, and bigger than a ten-gallon Stetson, it fit snugly atop the porcelain throne.

Not the place I usually hang my hat.

But the nurses said it was a very important accessory.

They used it as a yardstick to make sure my kidneys were still working properly after chemo.

The first time a nurse asked me if I'd tried the hat, I was a little confused. But then again, it was early in the morning and I wasn't fully awake yet.

"Did you void?"

"I'd love an Altoid.™"

That was pre-nausea.

During nausea, the only thing I consumed with any regularity was ice chips. Although, occasionally, one of the oncology nurses could get me to take a couple sips of hot chicken bouillon.

Oncology nurses are a wonderful thing.

The first nurse I had was a Princess Di look-alike named Jody. We loved her. She was sweet and kind and went out of her way to explain everything to us during my first chemo treatment—calming our fears and answering all our questions.

Then there was young Teresa, a newlywed from one of the Carolinas; can't remember whether it was North or South. I never was very good with directions.

Teresa was the tiniest little thing, but she had the biggest heart.

Whenever she gave me my medications, she always brought along an extra dose of compassion. When I had to throw up, she would hold the emesis basin and wipe my face with a cool cloth.

Ever wonder where the medical profession comes up with all these bizarre terms?

Emesis basin.

Sounds like a poet.

"And now, Emesis Basin will read to you from his collected works . . ."

Or suppository.

Another very literary-sounding term.

"Now, class, today we're going to suppose-a-story about . . ."

The first time a nurse had to give me a suppository I turned my head in embarrassment, which wasn't difficult since I had to turn on my side anyway. By my third treatment, suppositories were old hat. But I don't think the new male nurse shared my feelings.

It's amazing how rapidly one adjusts to the tenor of hospital life. Although it can become pretty boring after a while. There's not a whole lot you can do from bed.

I did manage to send out a record number of Christmas cards that year though. Since I could only write a few at a time before growing tired, I started in October. My friends and family all said it was the first time they'd ever received a Christmas card before Thanksgiving.

Like I said, boring.

I'd thought the hospital would be a great place to catch up on my reading, but the effort of holding a book, even my Bible, would exhaust me after only a few minutes.

So, in desperation, I turned to the boob tube instead.

Problem was, during the day there wasn't that big a selection. Since I've never been a fan of those screaming afternoon talk shows, soap operas became my pacifier.

It became a welcome diversion to immerse myself in the problems of the glamorous Erica Kane instead of wondering when I was going to throw up next.

I was fighting cancer.

Erica was fighting to keep control of her cosmetics empire.

I was fighting to keep the nausea at bay.

Erica was fighting the attraction to her latest love interest.

Nurse Teresa loved *All My Children*.

She would tape it during the day and watch it when she got home from work each night.

Sometimes, however, she couldn't wait to find out what happened so she'd come in my room and sneak a quick peek. Or if she was busy with another patient, she'd drop by later and ask, "What happened on our show today?"

There were times I'd miss "our show" if I had a visitor or was napping.

So the next day Teresa would fill me in.

"You'll never believe what Erica did!"

Soaps weren't my only diversion.

Friends dropped by to visit. The only problem was, I could never remember that they'd been there.

It's called chemo memory. Or rather, chemo memory loss.

For about three years after my last treatment, I used that excuse as my reason for forgetting anything. "Really? I don't remember saying/doing that. Must be the chemo." But the expiration date has passed on that excuse.

Now when I forget something, I just say, "must have had a menopause moment."

Not everyone has to be hospitalized overnight for their chemo treatments. In fact, most people don't. Instead, they get to go to a nice quiet outpatient room in a cancer center with oversized padded recliners where they lean back and "relax" during their treatment.

Barbara N. says when she goes for her chemo she always likes to talk to the people around her, since she's there for three or four hours at a time.

One day, the patient sitting in the chair next to Barbara said, "I just don't know what to eat. Everything makes me sick. Nothing tastes good to me."

Before Barbara had a chance to offer a suggestion, an older lady across the way piped up, "You need to eat some pickled pigs' feet, honey. They're so good."

Barbara's surprise must have shown on her face, because the woman then asked her, "*You* ever eat any pickled pigs' feet?"

"Well, er . . . no," said Barbara.

"You need to get the ones with the black label; you eat the knuckles and everything, num, num, num."

"The ones with the black label? Oh . . . okay."

Later when the pickled-pigs'-feet woman finished her treatment, she said over her shoulder to Barbara as she was leaving, "Now, honey, you make sure you get the ones with the black label."

Personally, I'm a little more partial to the black label that comes with See's truffles.

Not that I could have eaten pigs' feet *or* chocolate truffles in those days.

Besides, I don't think the hospital kitchen stocked either of those delicacies.

Ah, the hospital. Usually I had a three- to four-week break from it before I returned for my next chemo, but unfortunately, less than a week after my second treatment I was readmitted with a staph infection.

I was placed in an isolation room with the door kept tightly shut and signs posted everywhere saying "Use good handwashing" in an attempt to ward off further infection.

At least they didn't have to wash their feet.

It was nearly dusk one day when the door opened and a nurse I'd never seen before poked her head in and asked, "Mr. Walker, did you receive your flowers that were sent earlier?"

Granted, when she opened the door all she could see was a bald, makeup-less, flat-chested person sucking on a sponge-tipped mouth swab that probably looked like a lollipop.

So I can see how she might have mistaken me for a Kojak look-alike.

Until she heard me speak.

When she realized her faux pas, that poor nurse turned bright red, mumbled something about being in the wrong room, and beat a hasty retreat.

That never would have happened to Bonnie Sheaffer.

Whenever this elegant sixty-nine-year-old went in for her lounge chair chemo or radiation treatments, she was always well-dressed and wearing makeup. "It was very important for my own morale to put my face on and be neatly dressed," she said.

Guess I should have taken a few beauty tips from Bonnie.

A characteristic of the great saints is their power of levity. Angels can fly because they can take themselves lightly. One "settles down" into a sort of selfish seriousness; but one has to rise to a gay self-forgetfulness.
—G.K. Chesterton

six

What's Love Got to Do with It?

Everything. How the support of faith, family, and friends can make all the difference.

Love seeketh not itself to please,
Nor for itself hath any care,
But for another gives its ease,
And builds a Heaven in Hell's despair.
—WILLIAM BLAKE

A few days after my mastectomy when the hospital released me to go home, I wasn't quite at my movie-star best.

My hair was greasy, I hadn't had a bath or shower in three days (other than those quickie hospital sponge baths), I was lopsided, and I had a gross, plastic, football-shaped drainage tube under my arm filling up with icky bodily fluids.

That's when my best friend came over to visit and cheer me up.

Lana hugged me, gently, then wrinkled her petite little nose and said, "You stink."

"I love you too."

"We need to give you a bath."

Now Lana's five-foot-two and maybe 105 pounds. I'm five-foot-seven and haven't seen 105 since junior high. Plus I was still pretty sore from the surgery and not moving very easily.

Besides, Lana's no nurse.

But she teaches Special Ed.

And I think she must have written the manual on being a best friend.

It was wonderful to have my hair washed and feel all fresh and clean again. I'm not one of those wilderness women who can go a week or more without the porcelain amenities. Two days, tops. Two hours even better.

So I was very grateful for Lana's twelve-step bathing intervention.

Next she helped me don her gift of an oversized red shirt, which would cleverly disguise my flattened, bandaged chest, and a pair of perky canvas shoes. Lana's really into shoes. We call her the shoe queen; she has more shoes than Imelda Marcos.

The next step of her intervention was to get me outside in the fresh air for a walk. "We need to get you moving," she said briskly.

I never knew anyone so little could be so bossy.

And I could have taken her, I *know* I could have, but since I didn't want to rip out my stitches, I decided to wait for a better time.

Lana wasn't the only one who demonstrated unfailing love and support to me.

During the more than three months of intense chemo treatments, my family and Michael's family were both great—helping out in myriad practical ways.

Michael's sister Sheri did our laundry once a week, his sister-in-law Nancy hired a cleaning woman to clean our house, and his brother, Pastor Bob, chauffeured me to my doctor's appointments.

Hey, I could get used to this! Now, if I could only keep up my sick act a little longer . . .

I did.

And the chemo was a huge help in that regard. It effectively incapacitated me for a week or so after every treatment. I had no idea how weak and helpless those mega-chemo doses would leave me.

Not only does chemotherapy wipe out cancer cells, it also wipes out healthy, necessary cells that the body needs to function properly—including white and red blood cells. I became anemic due to a lack of healthy red blood cells.

And because red blood cells carry oxygen, my muscles, lungs, brain, and everything else in my body weren't getting enough oxygen to function correctly.

That's why after my second treatment, my oncologist cautioned me not to "do anything."

Guess my plans for painting the guest room and rearranging all the furniture would have to wait a while.

I didn't realize Dr. Caggiano meant "any" thing until I tried to make our bed, an important daily ritual to me. Okay, okay, since I know my mom and sister will be reading this, I cannot tell a lie. I admit it: *I don't always make the bed every day!* But on this particular day, a friend was coming over, and I didn't want her to see our messy, unmade bed.

I got as far as pulling up the sheet and blanket, but when I tried to pull up the heavy quilt, I collapsed in exhaustion on top of the covers.

Those extra heavy doses of chemo sapped all my energy. I became almost completely dependent on others to do things for me.

At least I could still go to the bathroom by myself.

But I had to plan the trip.

My aunt Sharon journeyed from Wisconsin to California to visit in between my treatments that November. She helped me decorate for Christmas while Michael was at work.

Actually, she decorated, and I directed. From the couch.

Sharon unpacked all the Christmas boxes and set the decorations on the floor in front of me so I could tell her where to put them: "The nativity goes on the mantel, the wreath goes on the door, and Michael's Father Christmas collection goes every place we can find room."

Next, Sharon unpacked the beautiful Victorian stocking Michael made me the year before—our first Christmas together. Now that man of mine can sew. He even surprised me with a thick terry cloth robe he'd made me—his first—as a welcome home gift from the hospital.

As Sharon oohed and aahed over the stocking, I came up with the brilliant idea to make *Michael* a stocking this year.

Only problem was, I didn't sew.

Neither did Aunt Sharon.

But we figured, how hard could it be?

So one day when I had a little more energy than usual, we drove to the fabric store and found some pre-quilted stocking panels. All I had to do was cut out on the dotted line and stitch around the sides.

Piece of fruitcake.

The cutting part went magnificently. Pinning it was a breeze. Then I lifted the little fabric-foot thingamajig on the sewing machine, inserted the stocking, pressed my foot on the pedal . . . and nothing happened.

Next, Sharon put pedal to the metal. Zilch.

After about twenty frustrating minutes of trying to make this lovingly handcrafted Christmas gift for my sweetie, I was ready to throw in the stocking and go buy him one instead.

That's when Sharon noticed a little button on the side of the machine.

The "on" switch.

Hey, how was I supposed to know? It was Michael's sewing machine, and as every wife knows, you don't mess with your husband's tools.

My tools were books.

In my B.C. (Before Cancer) days, I used to dream of staying home sick so I could lie in bed and read all day. During chemo, I thought those dreams had come true.

Unfortunately, the books were all too heavy for me. I'm not talking Solzhenitsyn or even the Brothers Grimm here. It was just that I was so weak, I didn't have the energy to even hold up the *TV Guide*.

So my brother-in-law Jim came to the rescue by loaning me his collection of James Bond movies. Once I made it through the whole *007* library, I started on our friend Carolyn's Elvis collection. *Viva Las Vegas!*

Amazing how a little Elvis and Sean Connery can perk up a girl's spirits.

Friends and family took turns coming over and staying with me since the doctor said I shouldn't be home alone, and Michael had already used up all his sick leave and vacation time.

One afternoon, Kim, a journalism pal from college, came over to keep me company. I asked if she could fix some lunch, but she's not too handy in the kitchen, so I had to coach her through the chicken noodle soup preparation.

"First you get the can opener . . ."

"What's it look like?"

My sister Lisa, a medical assistant at the time, volunteered to give me my daily GSF shots (granulocyte-colony stimulating factor), which helped my body replace the white blood cells that the chemo had destroyed.

The doctor said the shots needed to be given in the fatty parts of the body, so Lisa had a broad range of options.

One day she'd go for a thunder thigh, the next a little belly roll, and the next, my Bertha butt.

Even so, as time went on and my body became more stressed from the chemo, even the nerve endings in my skin were overloaded from the toxicity, so my body was sore everywhere.

The shots grew more and more painful until one night I screamed in pain.

Michael, my ever-protective hero, came running in demanding, "What did you do to my wife?!!"

He should have been more worried about my sister.

A couple weeks later, it was his turn to give me the shots since I'd just gotten over a staph infection, and my immune system was so compromised that we couldn't take the chance of anyone else coming into the house.

That's when I screamed at *him*.

Lucky guy. I'm sure at that moment he was really counting his marital blessings.

Those maternal blessings sure came in handy though.

My mom was a great comfort to me during this time because eight years earlier she'd had back-to-back—rather, chest-to-chest—mastectomies a year apart.

I'd always wanted to inherit something from my mom, but I'd sort of hoped it would be her size two genes rather than her tendency toward breast cancer.

However, knowing that she'd already been through the same thing and could understand how I felt was a big help. The simple fact that she'd survived this disease that had claimed other women's lives was an enormous encouragement to me.

When you're going through cancer, it helps tremendously to be around survivors.

It gives you hope.

At least it did for me.

My mom has always been one of my biggest champions. She's always believed in me, supported me, and thinks I can do anything.

Except math.

Friends can be supportive too.

Linda Gundy said that when she was going through chemo her best friend Cari wrote her a very special poem:

> *Roses are red*
> *Violets are tall*
> *I love you*
> *Bald head and all.*

Linda also has a beautiful journal her friend Judy made for her; it's filled with Scriptures of comfort, including:

> *Many are the afflictions of the righteous, but the*
> *LORD delivereth him out of them all.*
> —PSALM 34:19 KJV

Children can also be a great source of comfort.

Janis Whipple's three young nieces prayed daily for her hair to grow.

And Sherris White said that the kids in her son Samuel's kindergarten class all gathered around her one day, had her take off her hat, and prayed for her.

Kids do the sweetest things. Five-year-old Samuel also liked to pet his mom on her bald head. "I was like his little Chia pet," Sherris recalled.

Samuel preferred his mom without a wig.

Of course that might be because the day Sherris got her new hair she'd set it on a wig stand on the dresser in her bedroom. When Samuel came home from school, he went through her bedroom to use the bathroom and seconds later came running out crying: "There's somebody in your room with just a head, and his face is all white!"

Kids. Don't you love them? They really say the darndest things, as Art Linkletter long ago knew.

A few years after Beverly Pierce Stroebel had her mastectomy—in the late 1960s—she was in the shower one morning with her toddler, Jane.

Young Jane counted the nipples on her chest, then looked up at her mother's chest and asked, "Mommy, will I grow *one* like you, or *two* like my sisters?"

After the verb "To love," "To help" is the most beautiful verb in the world.

—Bertha Von Suttner

seven

Country Bear Jamboree Is Not a Rest Stop

Celebrating the end of chemotherapy with a trip
to Disneyland. I was looking for a rest stop,
he was looking for the rides.

*Make the best use of what is in your power, and
take the rest as it happens.*

—EPICTETUS

My husband is a Disnoid. The happiest place on earth is his favorite place on earth. He loves Splash Mountain, Pirates of the Caribbean, Tomorrowland, Fantasyland, Frontierland, and Whateverland.

But most of all, he loves Mickey. He does a great Mickey impression.

"There's a special feeling you get at Disneyland that you don't get anywhere else," Michael insists. Which is why he's visited the Magic Kingdom about a gazillion times. And why he was so eagerly looking forward to taking me someday—to share his favorite place in the world with his favorite person in the world (his words).

That day came in late December, a few weeks after my final chemotherapy treatment. We wanted to celebrate the end of chemo somehow, but our budget was pretty tight.

So Lana, my best friend who loves Mickey too, surprised us by announcing that she was taking us to Disneyland as a belated Christmas gift.

Michael was on cloud nine. I was pretty happy too—thrilled to be going *anywhere* away from hospitals, shots, and all-too-familiar bathrooms.

The morning of New Year's Eve found the three of us leaving Sacramento for the eight-hour drive to Southern California and the Magic Kingdom.

The first shock of the trip came when I pulled down the sun visor on my passenger side. As the late morning sun flooded the car with light, the mirror revealed something I hadn't noticed before: My eyebrows were completely gone!

I'd already been bald for a good three months, and others had noticed my lack of facial hair. In fact, I'd attended a Christmas party sporting a festive holiday scarf over my baldness and thinking I looked pretty good when an acquaintance I hadn't seen in some time blurted out through tear-filled eyes, "Oh, honey, you lost your eyebrows!"

"Eyelashes too," I said, smiling and batting my non-existent lashes to ease her discomfort. "In fact," I added as I leaned over and whispered in her ear, "I don't have a single hair *anywhere* on my body."

Now, *intellectually* I knew I didn't have eyebrows, I just didn't really KNOW it. When I looked in the mirror, I still *saw* my eyebrows—or rather, the indentation from where my eyebrows had been for thirty-some years. After living that long day-in and day-out with the same familiar face, you grow kind of accustomed to it and just see what you expect to see.

So I saw eyebrows.

It wasn't until the full morning sun was streaming in the car that I clearly saw for the very first time what everyone else had been seeing for months: My eyebrows were gone—vanished, vamoosed, nonexistent—and so were my eyelashes.

I looked like a refugee from another planet. The planet of no facial hair.

I burst into tears.

Talk about delayed reaction—*way* delayed. Okay, so call me oblivious.

How could I go out in public looking like that?

But my dear, ever-resourceful, take-charge friend Lana said that she'd just pencil in eyebrows and do my makeup and I'd look great.

The next morning we woke up bright and early so we could be at Disneyland the second those magic gates opened. It was a tad chilly so I wrapped a pretty silk scarf around my head, being careful not to cover the new eyebrows Lana had artfully sketched in, and then covered that with a cute denim cloche hat.

I was READY for Disneyland.

Or so I thought.

Since it was only ten days after my final chemo treatment, I was still pretty weak from the beating my body had taken over the past few months. My white count wasn't quite normal yet, so I had little energy and tired easily.

But one of the great things about the happiest place on earth is that they know how to treat their guests. Moments after arriving, we rented a wheelchair, and I rode in style all around the park. One wonderful, unexpected side benefit about being sick and in a wheelchair at Disneyland: There's no waiting in line. You get to go to the very front.

Cool.

Some teenagers evidently thought it was pretty cool too, because a little later, security caught them faking an injury to get wheelchair privileges. As the guards politely escorted them out of the line, I held my breath—and my hat—waiting to see if I'd be next; I was ready to remove my hat at a moment's notice if I needed to prove my illness authenticity.

They didn't ask.

The second shock of our trip came after we'd been at Disneyland just a few hours, and I casually asked, "So, will we be ready to leave after lunch?"

Michael and Lana both looked at me incredulously.

"You don't go to Disneyland for just a few hours," Michael said. "You stay until it closes."

"Until it closes?! What time is that?"

"Midnight."

"Midnight?!!! That's twelve more hours," I whined.

"Actually, Michael," Lana said, "I think I saw a sign that says the park closes early today because of the holiday."

Whew. Saved by the best friend.

"So what time *does* it close?" I asked.

"Ten P.M."

"*Ten* more hours?! What are we going to *do* for all that time?"

Lana and Michael exchanged more incredulous glances.

To them—and every other Disnoid—the only way to *do* Disneyland is arrive the minute the gates open and stay until they close fifteen hours later.

But I wasn't a Disnoid. So to me, you go in, ride a few rides, see a few shows, buy an overpriced tourist memento from one of the shops, eat a corndog and some cotton candy, ride a couple more rides, and head home.

Five or six hours. Tops.

Can you say failure to communicate?

Things got a little tense there for a few minutes, until I figured out a happy solution. "I know! Let's go to the bookstore; I'll find a good book or a couple magazines and just sit and read for a few hours while you guys go on more rides," I suggested brightly.

"There's no reading at Disneyland!" Michael sputtered.

Not only was there nowhere in all of Disneyland to buy the latest best-seller—yes, they sell books, but I wasn't in the mood for *Mickey and the Beanstalk*—but even if there had been, there was still another major problem: no place to just sit and read. A huge amusement park deficiency as far as I was concerned.

Huge.

I may have had my own chair, but there was no quiet warm place to park it.

Granted, there are plenty of restaurants with indoor seating. But, just like all the rides, there's always a waiting line to get in.

So much for lingering over a nice cup of tea and a book.

You would think the Magic Kingdom of all places would have somewhere to enjoy a spot of tea. After all, they have that teacup ride.

Now I was starting to get a little bit crabby. It really was a small world after all, and that world was quickly closing in on me.

W-a-a-a-a-g-h!!

Lucky Lana and Michael. At that moment I'm sure they felt they'd just met the eighth dwarf—Whiny.

Not wanting to ruin the day for them, however, I suggested we go on some more rides, which I loved—particularly Star Tours. The problem was, the rides only lasted three or four minutes, and afterwards, the day still stretched interminably before us.

So we went shopping.

Michael got a Mickey mug, Lana got a Mickey mug, and I got a pretty pearl bracelet—minus any Disney figures.

Four hours and counting.

We used up another hour with dinner, but by that time Whiny was fast becoming Sleepy.

All I wanted was a little nap. But since Disneyland doesn't have any nap rides, I asked Michael and Lana to park me in the lobby of Country Bear Jamboree for an hour or so where I could catch some z's while they rode some more rides.

They hesitated, but I assured them I'd be just fine. I also hinted that by the time they returned, Whiny might have metamorphosed into Happy.

They were out of there in a Space Mountain second.

I settled in for a nice little catnap in a corner of the lobby, but just as I began to nod off, the doors to the Bear Auditorium swung open to let in a new round of laughing, sometimes crying, children and their parents. Little did I know that those Jamboree doors would swing open every twelve minutes letting out and taking in a new batch of kids each time while piping out the same tune over and over again—"It's a small world, after all; it's a small world . . ."

Oops. Wrong attraction. I wasn't in Fantasyland. Or even slumberland.

Unfortunately.

The day did end on a high note with Fantasmic. Wow! Pretty amazing stuff. Enough to make me forget my tiredness. And once again my illness opened magic doors for us: We got a seat up front on a roped-off portion of the lawn reserved for people—and their families—in wheelchairs.

Yet as much as I loved Fantasmic, I didn't love it enough to put in a twelve- to fifteen-hour day at the park. The next time we do Disneyland, we're staying at the Disneyland Hotel, so I can ride the monorail back for some essential reading and nap time.

We may just have to switch over to the Disneyland Pacific Hotel instead though, because I've just learned that in the afternoons they now hold a *Practically Perfect Tea with Mary Poppins* in a lovely Victorian garden room.

Now that's more my cup of tea.

Book 'em, Mickey.

> *Let me not to the marriage of true minds*
> *Admit impediments.*
>
> —WILLIAM SHAKESPEARE

eight

Single Women, Single Breasts

The unique challenges single women face after "losing" one (or both) breasts.

I will lie down and sleep in peace,
for you alone, O LORD,
make me dwell in safety.

—PSALM 4:8

When Lynda Duncan went to her twenty-fifth high school reunion as a single woman she preferred to hear about her classmates' lives rather than talk about hers.

But after two and a half decades, her classmates wanted an update.

So she said, "You want to hear about what I do for a living, what I do for personal fulfillment, my conversion to Christianity, my topless video, or my seven tattoos?"

Then Lynda would look at her friends with a total deadpan expression and easily turn the conversation back to them.

If pressed for an explanation, however, she'd answer, "Uncle Sam pays the bills because I work for the government; I work with high school students for personal fulfillment; my conversion was in 1979; the topless video was because I came through radiation so well that the doctors wanted to do a topless and headless video to visually demonstrate the lack of negative impact of the radiation—no burning or scarring; and the seven tattoos were for radiation treatment."

Lynda is a breast cancer survivor.

So is Janis Whipple, who was thirty-four and also single when she was diagnosed. Although her cancer was discovered in only one breast, due to its aggressive nature, Janis opted for a bilateral mastectomy followed by immediate reconstructive surgery.

When her plastic surgeon came in to check on her the day after her surgery, he asked, "Is there anything I can get for you?"

Without missing a beat, Janis replied, "Yeah, a cute young doctor would be nice."

Some men are a little intimidated to ask this book editor and former public relations director with a Master of Arts from Southern Baptist Theological Seminary for a date. "You add The Big C to that, especially breast cancer, and it kind of made me feel like here's another big dating strike against me," she said.

"In fact," Janis added with a laugh, "two strikes."

But now, she doesn't think it will be an issue with a man she would date at this time in her life. "The idea of having to deal with that still sometimes scares me," she said, "but I also believe that it's not fair of me to prejudge someone whom I haven't even met yet."

Beverly Ann, who was forty-one when she was diagnosed, said going through breast cancer as a single person didn't bother her. "I know a lot of married people feel sorry for us single women," she said. "They think we must have it difficult, when in fact it is probably easier for us to make decisions about treatments when we're single."

When Beverly was home and didn't feel good, she would just lie down.

She didn't cook.

She didn't clean.

She didn't talk.

I was neck-and-neck with her on the first two out of three.

But not talking? That's like asking me not to breathe.

"I was very blessed during my treatment," Beverly recalls. "The Lord and my mom were always there for me."

One way Beverly's mom helped was by cooking all her favorite foods.

The only problem was, the food was so good that Beverly gained about forty pounds after the surgery over an eight-month period. She'd initially lost eighteen pounds before the surgery due to nerves. "My family and I started eating the day I got out of the hospital," she said.

"Since I hadn't eaten in the hospital, I was hungry, so I asked my folks to stop at Burger King on the way home, where I got a Double Whopper, king size fries, and double chocolate shake figuring I would never be able to eat it. Surprise! I just kept eating, waiting to get sick, which never happened.

"My surgeon said I could eat anything I wanted. Well, I ate everything. All my lifetime favorites. Foods I had not eaten for years! It was wonderful."

Janis also gained some weight during her treatments.

"I figured if I didn't know how long I was going to have, I was going to eat all the McDonald's French fries I wanted," she said with a laugh.

What Janis didn't have was the in-the-same-town support of her very close family; she lived in Nashville and her family members were living in Florida at the time.

"That's when it was hard to be single," she said.

Geography couldn't prevent her loved ones from staying in constant touch and daily prayer for Janis however. Additionally, each member of her family took turns coming out to stay with her for a week at a time during the surgery, subsequent treatments, and hospitalizations. "It was great," Janis said. "I have a really close family and they were here for me, but when the last person in my family left and no one was coming back, that was difficult."

She admits that although she felt vulnerable at that time, there was also a part of her that needed to be alone.

Janis was never totally alone though. Her best friend Kelly was in steadfast attendance during all her surgeries, treatments, and hospitalizations.

A couple years after her double mastectomy, doctors found a recurrence of cancer in Janis's sternum, so she then had to undergo radiation, chemo, a stem-cell transplant, and more chemo.

"Kelly would be there to hold my hand, pray, and take me for walks in the corridors. She even bought me a pair of bunny slippers to wear in the hospital, and she had a pair herself she would wear with me on our walks," Janis recalled.

"I could not have gone through my experiences—being single—without her love, support, and just her presence," she added. "I knew it wouldn't matter what I did, said, or looked like, she would be there."

God was always there for Janis too. One of the many Scripture passages that sustained her during this time was:

> *"Because he loves me," says the LORD, "I will*
> *rescue him;*
> *I will protect him. . . .*
> *He will call upon me, and I will answer him;*
> *I will be with him in trouble,*
> *I will deliver him and honor him.*
> *With long life will I satisfy him and show him*
> *my salvation."*
> —PSALM 91:14–16

Then there were the friends and coworkers who demonstrated their love through action. "People cut my grass, fed my dog, and stocked my freezer with food; one friend even came and cleaned my house for me," she said.

As a busy book editor, member of her church worship team, and Bible study leader, Janis was accustomed to wearing many hats. She just didn't realize she'd amass such a large quantity—nearly ninety altogether.

Janis recalls one time during the summer when she and her family went to San Francisco to see her brother perform in a vocal competition. Since she was wearing a hat, her whole family wore hats too, for solidarity. "They carried their hats all the way from Florida in their suitcases just for me," she said.

It wasn't only her family who tipped their hats to Janis.

During the chemo months, she usually wore a hat to work every day. One day when Janis arrived at the office, she noticed a couple guys wearing baseball caps inside the building, but she didn't think much about it.

Then when she checked her e-mail there was a message from a coworker—one whom she didn't even know that well—who had organized "hat day" as a show of encouragement to Janis.

"I walked into a morning meeting, and everyone had hats on," she recalled. And when she went to the cafeteria at lunchtime, many people were also wearing hats—everything from nurse's caps and paper hats to vintage Air Force helmets.

Janis had her picture taken with the cafeteria-hat brigade. It now proudly hangs in her cubicle at work.

Wigs and hats aren't the only thing women need to adjust to during and after breast cancer.

When Beverly, an African American, first went to get fitted for her breast prosthesis, she asked the saleswoman if it came in a variety of skin colors.

"The clerk said, 'Yeah, but no one's going to see it,'" Beverly recalled.

Beverly's response?

"Well, *I'm* going to see it!"

She's quite happy her prosthesis comes in her skin tone. "That way if I wear a lacy bra," Beverly explained, "the brown still shows through."

Beverly is now a volunteer with the American Cancer Society and tries to support other women going through breast cancer—including her own cousin.

According to the American Cancer Society, African-American women are more likely to die of breast cancer than are women of any other racial or ethnic group. Yet only 54.9 percent of African-American women over the age of fifty report having had a mammogram and a clinical breast exam within the previous two years.

Beverly notes that, with the exception of her mom, her friends and family who are women of color do not talk much about such things. "I would like to see that change and am making an effort to help that," Beverly said.

Janis Whipple's mom was also helpful to her and gave her some great words of wisdom. "She reminded me that I didn't need to be around anyone who was negative during the process."

So Janis made a few new friends.

Okay, they were wigs, but she named them.

Loretta she met through the mail.

She was a wig without a name when Janis first spotted her in a mail-order catalog, but once that headless hairpiece arrived in Nashville and Janis and her best friend saw that BIG hair up close and personal, they christened her Loretta.

Although they don't have too much in common, Loretta has happily accompanied Janis to a couple costume parties.

After Loretta, Janis's doctor wrote her a prescription for another wig.

"He called it a 'cranial prosthesis' and I thought, 'Just what I need, a new brain.'"

Janis had five wigs altogether, and she named them all: Pam, Susie, Nancy, Tammy, and of course, Loretta.

There is a friend who sticks closer than a brother.
—Proverbs 18:24

nine

Humorous Tales from the Front

Or what happens when your bra "stuffing" travels to the center of your chest during an important business meeting.

Laughter is by definition healthy.

—Doris Lessing

I don't know about you, but when I gain weight, my breasts get fuller. And when I lose weight, they're the first things to go.

Naturally, once I got "healthy" again, I regained all the weight I'd lost during chemo—and then some. So my real breast got bigger. But the new-and-improved rebuilt one didn't.

See the problem?

You got it. Lopsided.

I had quite a difficult time finding bras to fit. Actually, I never did find a bra that fit just right. So for years I kept stuffing the cups with everything imaginable—tissue, toilet paper, shoulder pads, my husband's quilt batting—whatever worked.

With varying degrees of success.

Toilet paper was okay, but it didn't have the same puffy volume that tissues had.

One or two tissues didn't do anything at all while five or six tended to leave a noticeable bulge—especially when I was wearing T-shirts. I finally settled on four tissues as the perfect number.

But it wasn't an infallible solution. So I tried to disguise my uneven chest as best I could by wearing loose-fitting tops or by layering with vests or funky jackets.

Who says the Annie Hall look is out of style?

Although I did have to upgrade it a couple years later when I was working as a writer in the marketing department of a small, private, upscale company complete with cook and a workout facility.

Classy stuff.

My boss—the marketing manager—was also pretty classy and just a tad intimidating. She was tall, blonde, slender, always perfectly coifed, immaculately dressed in subtle understated designer clothes (think beige and cream), and brilliant at her job.

As a former low-paid reporter for a weekly community newspaper who usually shopped the sales racks at the nearest discount stores, I felt a little out of my league.

During our weekly marketing meeting, we'd report on our projects and bring everyone up-to-date. One day my boss said she'd like me to give a special presentation of my project the following week.

The night before the meeting I was pretty nervous—going over my notes again and again to make sure I was prepared and carefully selecting the right outfit to wear: professional but not too formal, confident yet comfortable.

I walked into the meeting a little apprehensively, but as my presentation successfully progressed, I relaxed. Suddenly, I had an uncontrollable need to scratch, in a very inappropriate, unprofessional place—between my breasts.

As I glanced down, I discovered the reason why.

Peeking out over the top of my white V-necked blouse was the polyester quilt batting I'd stuffed in my bra that morning to compensate for my uneven look. Unbeknownst to me, because I have no feeling on my reconstructed breast side, the very itchy batting had traveled to the middle of my chest during the meeting.

Faster than the flipping of a chart, I turned my back on my colleagues—under the guise of illustrating a point on the white board—and surreptitiously tucked the batting back down inside my bra, stealing a quick scratch in the process.

They never noticed a thing.

Once the meeting concluded, I hurried to the bathroom where I pulled out the offending polyester batting and replaced it with the soothing natural fibers of toilet paper.

After this embarrassing incident, I thought I should perhaps try something a little more stationary.

Since Michael's pretty handy with a needle, and I'm not, he decided to lend his talents to the problem. We went to a fabric store to buy shoulder pads, which he planned to sew inside my bra.

They came two in a package, so when we got home I tried the double-stuffed look, but now I was *really* off-kilter—the other way. So we settled for less-is-more, thinking that did the trick.

It didn't.

Yet I didn't realize it until many months later when I saw myself in a photo taken with my two closest friends.

Can you say leaning tower of Pisa?

When I showed the photo to my mom and bemoaned my lopsided look, she suggested that I have the doctor write me a prescription for a prosthesis.

"I won't qualify. I've already had reconstructive surgery," I lamented.

"Have you asked?" she countered. Ever notice that no matter how old you get, your mother's always a mother?

I made an appointment with my doctor for a week later. She promptly wrote me a prescription for a "mastectomy bra" or prosthesis to even me out.

With prescription in hand, I visited a specialty boutique where a saleswoman fitted me with a silicone prosthesis that looks and feels remarkably like a real breast, complete with simulated nipple "bump."

She told me I could either wear the prosthesis inside the pocket of my new mastectomy bra or simply molded against my skin and held in place by the bra. The latter looked a bit more real, and since I'm all for feeling like a natural woman, I left it plastered to my chest.

It was great. For the first time in years, my breasts matched!

I love my new prosthesis so much that I even wear it around the house on weekends—times that I usually go braless.

The first Saturday I wore it, we had a plumber come to the house to replace a broken toilet. While he was intently removing the toilet bolts, I was scrubbing away vigorously at some hard water stains in the bathtub.

Suddenly we both heard it.

SPLAT.

We looked down. There, balanced remarkably on the edge of the bathtub, sat my new prosthesis in all its quivering pink glory.

"Oops; lost my breast," I said, casually scooping up the silicone before his astonished eyes.

"It's new," I added as if that explained everything.

His eyes widened even more when I nonchalantly stuffed the prosthesis back down inside my shirt and resumed my scrubbing.

Good thing the plumber's married to my best friend.

Give me a sense of humor, Lord;
Give me the grace to see a joke,
To get some happiness from life,
And pass it on to other folk.
—Prayer in Chester Cathedral

ten

Her Body, His Pain

His fear and pain that are often overlooked
in the midst of her disease—a revealing look
at how husbands cope.

Grow old along with me! The best is yet to be.
—Robert Browning

A woman's breast cancer doesn't affect only the woman. It also strongly impacts the man who loves her. In many ways, I think the experience is much harder on him, partly because he feels so powerless. Men are great "fixers." But this is something they can't fix. What they can do—hopefully—is love, support, and reassure you.

And tell you you're beautiful. That's a biggie.

But I digress. This is Michael's story. Take it away, honey.

Michael's Story

Laura's asked me to share a little about my side of the story—what it's like to go through breast cancer from the husband's point of view.

To be completely honest, it stinks. Especially when you're a newlywed.

I had long heard that the first year of marriage is usually difficult. Even more so when the couple gets married later in life. But knowing this, we were able to avoid many of the pitfalls and our first year was, actually, great.

Sure, there were major adjustments—and major head-butting sessions.

After all, we were both in our thirties and strong, independent individuals with artistic temperaments. But things were going well. Life was anew with possibilities, and our first anniversary was wonderful.

Then there was the biopsy.

Throughout the procedure, I was completely unaware anything was wrong. In my naiveté, this was all just routine, so I wasn't the least bit worried.

Then the surgeon came into the room where my mother-in-law and I were waiting; she was concerned because the lump looked "unusual."

The pathologist confirmed her suspicions.

Cancer.

I was blindsided.

Mom and I held Laura's hands when the doctor broke the news to my beloved: "I'm afraid it was cancerous."

I remember wanting to jump in and buffer the news. This was too straightforward. Too blunt. How was my bride going to respond?

Laura started to cry, and Mom embraced her. I don't remember what I did, but somehow I got the signal that mother and daughter needed time alone together. So I walked into the waiting room.

Needing to do something, I phoned my sister, Sheri.

Ten years my senior, Sheri had always been a kind of mom to me. We've always been close, and it was she whom I turned to for comfort. It wasn't until I said the word *cancer* that I began to fall apart.

Sheri knows me better than anyone else on earth—in fact, at that early stage in my marriage, she knew me even better than Laura did.

And she knew what I needed to hear.

"You pull it together!" she challenged in a firm, authoritative voice. "Your wife needs you right now. You fall apart *later,* away from Laura. She needs your strength and needs you to be there for her now."

I doubt any human being could have said anything to me at that moment that was more appropriate or more needed. I firmly believe that God inspired every word Sheri said to me during that telephone conversation.

It was my call to action.

I don't remember whose idea it was, but I determined that Laura would not see my doubts, my fears, my weakness. I would receive my support elsewhere and would be nothing but supportive and encouraging to Laura.

Little did I understand what this would mean, but it gave me a mission and a purpose. And it set into motion the role I was to play over the next several months.

I became Laura's primary caregiver, changing her IV bags, giving her shots, and making sure the nursing staff gave her medicines on time. I learned more than any layperson should ever have to know about medications.

I tried not to feel. Anything.

I tried just to be. To do. To make it through one moment at a time and face each challenge as it arose.

During the mastectomy and first chemo treatment, I did quite well, if I do say so myself. At least on the outside. Most of the wonderful knight-in-shining-armor stories Laura tells about me happened during this period.

Then there's the rest of the story.

After they put the chemotherapy into Laura's body for the first time, I went for a "walk." Laura didn't find out until much later that I went in search of a place where I could throw up. I had never faced anything so difficult as watching someone put something lethal into the woman I loved. And being totally powerless to do anything about it.

While I was able to successfully function, I was in denial of my feelings. I was not dealing with what was really going on inside me.

Many were the times I froze upon entering Laura's room while she was sleeping. My own breath stopped until I confirmed that her breath continued. Deep below the surface, I was terrified I might lose her.

And the anger grew little by little.

Yes, at first I held the bucket while Laura threw up. Not glamorous, but I was after all in "function" mode. After the second treatment, I would bring her a cool cloth and put it on the back of her neck while she vomited. After the third treatment, I called into the bathroom to be sure she was okay.

But after the last treatment, I would get up and move to the other end of the house when she retched.

I couldn't deal with it anymore.

A lot of it simply had to do with my being progressively worn down. But also, each session got worse and worse for Laura and therefore also for me.

I was working my full-time, stressful job by day and taking care of Laura throughout the night. Once, after she was hospitalized with a cold, I asked most of our friends and family not to visit because her immune system was weak and the risk of infection too great.

This meant I had even more work to do.

I had a meltdown in front of my sister. The pent-up anger erupted, and I began yelling about how unfair everything was. "I didn't buy into this!" I spewed.

"Yes you did," came Sheri's gentle reply. "I heard you. For better, for worse. In sickness and in health."

Wow.

Sure, it was true that this was unfair.

Unfair to Laura that she had cancer.

Unfair to me that I had to give her shots and wake up every two hours to change IV bags.

Unfair that this should happen so early in our marriage.

But so what?

"Stuff happens" (my paraphrase) became one of my main philosophies.

I could never believe that my loving God would *cause* the cancer. And I still refuse to believe that God would *want* us to go through this. Laura got cancer because "stuff" happens.

Period.

God never promised us that life would be fair. Just the opposite. In this life we will have trials and tribulations.

God did, however, promise that He would cause good to come out of bad, and I clung to that. It didn't alleviate the anger, but it helped me cope.

The days went by, and the chemo sessions ended. The IV tubes and the shots were discontinued, and Laura slowly recovered.

Strangely, my anger turned into depression, a depression that lasted several months. For the longest time I didn't know why. Then it hit me. Laura didn't *need* me anymore.

I had been her caregiver, her nurse, her protector. But now she was able to do things for herself again. I felt I had no identity.

I knew that the cancer had irrevocably changed me, that I would never be the same again. And now the person I became during treatment was no longer necessary.

As Laura began to put her life back in order, my life was lost at sea. It took me over a year to recover emotionally, partly because I didn't open up to anyone.

And even now there are wounds that are still tender. To this day, I cannot be within earshot of Laura when she's throwing up. *Love you, but you're on your own, babe.*

A few years ago, my coworker Jonie's sister was diagnosed with ovarian cancer, and Jonie became one of her primary caregivers. Because our desks were next to each other, we talked frequently about what was going on. I was amazed at the parallels between Laura and the sister, and also between Jonie and me. Even down to the "who-am-I-now" lostness when her sister became self-sufficient again. In sharing my story, I helped Jonie. I was able to listen and empathize because I had been there, done that.

In many ways, I am a private person. My preference would be to put all this behind us. There is a part within me that dreads pulling up the past and reliving that period in our lives. But that's not what life, what God, has in store for us.

Soon after Laura's hair grew back, she wrote her cancer story for our local newspaper. My aunt Betty, who works in a doctor's office, recounted a story she'd heard from the office nurse. One of their patients knew she had a lump in her breast, but she was so afraid, she wouldn't come in and have it checked. Then she read the newspaper story and told the nurse that, as a result, she decided if that woman's husband (moi) was supportive, perhaps she needn't fear her own husband's reaction. So she made the appointment.

I was amazed. It was my supporting Laura that helped this woman overcome her fear.

We were given a gift of hearing about someone touched by the article. The woman was simply sharing with her nurse, not knowing that my aunt—who was related to the writer—worked in that office. The nurse shared it with Betty, who shared it with us.

Earlier, I mentioned the promise that God causes all things to work together for good. The good coming out of Laura's cancer is that she—and I, to a small degree—have been able to help and comfort so many others.

Each spring and fall, I volunteer for American Cancer Society fund-raisers. I share with friends and strangers—both men and women—about mammograms and mastectomies.

It is part of who I have become.

Not too long ago I walked past a female coworker and noticed she was crying. We sometimes get trying phone calls at work, so I made a comment about "getting beaten up by another customer." She replied she wished it was only that. She had just gotten the results of her mammogram.

Instantly, I told her we were going outside to talk.

Once outside, I asked for details. There was a "mass" and the doctor's office wanted her to come back in for an ultrasound. She heard the word *mass* and thought of some huge thing growing inside her and was afraid it was going to kill her.

Now I've come a long way from those early marital days when buying "feminine products" for Laura embarrassed me.

I mean, I'm a man. Talking to a woman who is not my wife, mother, or sister, about something growing inside her breast—does this seem at all weird? It did to her husband, who knew me in high school.

And sometimes it does to me too.

But in this instance, I was able to talk logically to her. Right then, fear was her greatest enemy. Fear was clouding her ability to reason. Once we worked through some of the fear, half the battle was won. I was able to encourage her to fight the fear with knowledge.

Because of what Laura and I had gone through, I was equipped to share information. *Mass* doesn't necessarily refer to size but is just another word for *thing* or *growth*. We talked for several minutes, and when we returned to our desks, she was greatly relieved.

Demystifying the unknown.

As it turned out, she's fine. The mass was benign.

I'll say it again: God promised He would bring good from the bad. Because I had been there, I was able to bring comfort to someone who was hurting.

Good. God's good.

There's nothing funny about cancer—for the patient or a loved one. It's not funny, it's terrifying.

So what should you do? Be a frightened spectator? We say not. Humor is a very powerful ally in the battle, and Laura and I laughed a lot, especially in the beginning.

It helped us through the really tough times to come.

And then, the day Laura finished the last of her reconstructive surgery, her car was stolen out of our driveway while we were at the surgery center.

When we arrived home and discovered this, we laughed. And laughed. After all we'd been through, that this should happen that day of all days was absurd. Sometimes if you don't laugh, you'll cry.

We chose laughter.

> *But those who suffer he delivers in their suffering;*
> *he speaks to them in their affliction.*
>
> —Job 36:15

eleven

I'll Show You Mine If You'll Show Me Yours

Sharing with other women helps diffuse the fear of The Big C.

You don't live in a world all alone.
Your brothers are here too.
—ALBERT SCHWEITZER

The first person I ever knew who had breast cancer was my great-aunt Annette. "Aunt" Annette is my grandpa Augie's niece, so if you want to be particular, she's really my second cousin. But cousins are for roller-skating, sleepovers, and kick-the-can. And I've never kicked-the-can with Aunt Annette. Besides, have you ever tried explaining to a nine-year-old that a grown-up more than three times her age is her cousin?

And so, Aunt Annette she's stayed.

Aunt Annette was diagnosed with breast cancer when she was forty-two. She's now seventy-eight and has been cancer-free for nearly four decades.

"It didn't bother me from when I first found out about it," she said. "To me, it's not an arm or a leg. Besides, I only weigh eighty-eight pounds, so whether I have a bra on or not, nobody knows."

A couple years after Annette's surgery the girls' gym teacher from the local high school was planning to talk to her students about the importance of doing breast self-exams. She asked my aunt if she would come to school and share her breast cancer experience with the class.

She did—happily.

Aunt Annette advised the girls to do a breast self-exam every month after their period.

Then she turned her back to them briefly, adding when she turned around, "Otherwise, you're going to have this kind of a problem," and she threw her prosthesis up in the air and caught it.

Talk about a visual aid.

Then there's physical therapist Barbara Johnson, who'd had a really rough time during her breast cancer experience. Upon her return to work as a supervisor, her staff of thirty-plus physical and occupational therapists—male and female—were full of concern and questions.

Lots of questions.

So, during her first weekly staff meeting, Barbara matter-of-factly reached inside her blouse, pulled out her prosthesis, and set it on the table.

Time for show-and-tell.

What a great way to alleviate fears and demystify the unknown. However, I don't think that particular demonstration would have gone over quite as well at say Hewlett-Packard or IBM.

I've done the prosthesis presentation on occasion myself, sometimes even on purpose. But not always. (As you now know.)

And I've also flashed my rebuilt breast now and again, especially when it was brand-spanking new, but only to women. It's kind of like showing off your remodeled home to friends and family once the construction's finally complete.

There's a great sense of relief—and pride—in the final product.

Anyone who's ever done any remodeling or extensive home improvement projects knows how important it is to maintain a sense of humor during the ongoing construction.

That's why during one woman's reconstruction her teenage daughter made her assorted "pasties" to wear on her breast-in-progress. When the doctor opened her gown he was greeted by a smiley face.

Smiley face notwithstanding, not everyone's ready to see surgery scars and rebuilt breasts.

I remember visiting my girlfriend at the beauty salon where she worked just a few days before my mastectomy. One of her customers—who'd already had plastic reconstructive breast surgery—arrived for her appointment, so my friend introduced us and told her I'd be having the same surgery soon.

Before I had a chance to even blink, this fiftyish woman I'd never seen before in my life lifted up her shirt and flashed me!

"Isn't it great?" she beamed proudly. "My plastic surgeon did a wonderful job."

"Um, yeah . . . nice," I stammered, looking past her nervously at the wide-open front door of the shop.

I'm more of a behind-closed-doors, show-my-new-breast-to-people-I-know kind of person.

So's my mom. In fact, she likes to keep things all in the family.

A year or so after Mom's second mastectomy, my eleven-year-old niece (her granddaughter), Letitia, was visiting from Phoenix.

Letitia's always been very frank and curious, so she had a million questions to ask her grandma about breast cancer, her surgery, treatment, and recovery.

And she really wanted to know what the "pretend" breast looked like.

So Mom removed her prosthesis and let her granddaughter examine it.

"It feels just like a real one!" Letitia exclaimed.

Next, Mom showed Letitia her mastectomy scars and said, "See; I'm flat-chested like you were a year ago." (My niece was an early bloomer.)

"Grandma, that doesn't matter," Letitia said. "You're still living. That's what's important."

Out of the mouths of babes . . .

Artist Eve Dorf, who was forty-nine when she was diagnosed, found another visual way to share with other women—and men—what it's like to go through breast cancer.

She painted.

"A friend of mine suggested I put my feelings down on paper, so that's what I did," she said. "Whenever I came home depressed or tired from one of my chemo or radiation treatments I sat down and did a small painting."

At an art exhibit a couple years ago, I had the privilege of seeing Eve's "small" paintings, which chronicled her feelings during her treatments.

They made me weep.

Especially "Crocodile Tears," which showed a bald Eve crying the day she visited a wig shop. Every woman who's lost her hair to chemo can relate to that.

But her twenty beautiful watercolors and acrylics also included some whimsical paintings too, such as "Happy Face" and "The Bride Liked My Hat."

What began as therapy for Eve now continues to help hundreds of women as her exhibit makes the rounds of various hospitals, cancer centers, and art galleries.

Aunt Annette has helped countless women as well.

When she had her surgery in the mid '60s, it was only the third time her doctor had performed a mastectomy. She also had a hysterectomy during the same hospital stay; back then, the medical profession thought the two were related, since they were both "female problems."

Shortly after Annette's recovery, her doctor called and asked if she'd go talk to another woman who'd been recently diagnosed and was frightened by the prospect of surgery.

Aunt Annette did. And then a few months later she talked to another woman.

And another.

And another.

Since then she can't recall the number of women she's visited and talked with over the years about breast cancer.

Today there's a breast cancer support group that meets at St. Mary's Hospital in Racine, Wisconsin, on the third Saturday of each month thanks to my Aunt Annette who started it, one woman at a time, many years ago.

Whoever is happy will make others happy too.

—ANNE FRANK

twelve

I Will Never Leave You or Forsake You

Confronting the not-so-funny fear of dying, at 3 A.M.,
alone in my hospital bed.

There are times in a man's life when, regardless of the attitude of the body, the soul is on its knees in prayer.
—Victor Hugo

My friend Debbie was forty-three when she was diagnosed with breast cancer. A pastor's wife with two children, she has walked with the Lord since she was a child of ten.

But that didn't stop her from feeling fear when she faced the prospect that she might die from the cancer.

When she brought home a stack of chemotherapy brochures from the oncologist and she and her husband read about all the potential risks and side effects, she remembers asking, "Why would you even want to go on? Wouldn't you be better off just dying?

"As I was saying that, I suddenly realized I could die," she recalled. "Don and I were facing that together, and he was saying 'I don't want you to die . . .'"

At that instant the phone rang. It was Debbie's sister-in-law who had just heard the news. She was calling to tell Debbie not to take on everyone else's chemo horror stories as her own—at the very same time that Don and Debbie were reading various chemo horror stories.

"That wasn't a coincidence," Debbie says. "That was God saying to me he cared what I was going through at that very moment, and he was there with me. He was telling me, 'Don't worry, I've got you in my hands.'"

Later in her cancer experience Debbie remembers praying that if she were to die, God would prepare a mother and a wife to replace her.

"I wanted that person to be prepared and my kids to be accepting of her," she recalled. She was very practical and dry-eyed as she wrote to the Lord in her journal: "I want you to prepare someone else to take my place who would be even better than I was."

As she recounts the story to me now, however, the memory brings tears to her eyes.

But happily, she and her family haven't had to discover whether there's another woman who could fill her shoes or their hearts. She continues to fill both very nicely.

After her surgery, when she was hurting and depressed, Debbie thought about death. "It's real tempting to dwell on the negative parts when you're recovering and you're wondering if there is any light at the end of the tunnel," she said.

I can certainly relate to that feeling—especially the light at the end of the tunnel part.

I'll never forget one incident a couple days after my third chemo treatment.

I was sleeping in the guest bedroom at the front of the house near the bathroom, hooked up to my portable IV. Getting up in the middle of the night to go to the bathroom I was suddenly hit with a spasm of dry heaves. I made it to the toilet bowl, but there was nothing in my stomach to throw up.

As I headed back to the bedroom pushing the IV in front of me across the loud hardwood floor, another spasm assaulted me, doubling me over in its intensity.

Followed by another. And another.

Sinking to the hard floor, I prayed for death. "Lord, just take me now; I can't take any more. It's too much."

Weak and spent, I fell asleep on the floor.

Twenty minutes later I crawled back to bed and slept through the rest of the night without any further attacks.

Throughout most of my cancer ordeal, people kept marveling at my "good attitude" and wondered how I could stay so positive and upbeat during the experience.

The answer is God.

The other answer is, they didn't see me that lonely, terrifying night at 3 A.M. in the hospital following my second chemotherapy treatment when I fearfully confronted the very real possibility that I might die.

Even though Michael was asleep on a hospital cot right next to my bed, I didn't want to wake him, because as much as he loves me, I knew that he couldn't prevent death from claiming me.

I'd never felt so alone. Or so scared.

Frantically, I grabbed my Bible from the nightstand and started paging through it as I inwardly cried out to God, "Help me, help me."

He did. With the words of Psalm 18:

137

The cords of death entangled me;
the torrents of destruction
overwhelmed me.
The cords of the grave coiled around me;
the snares of death confronted me.
In my distress I called to the Lord;
I cried to my God for help. . . .

He reached down from on high and
took hold of me;
he drew me out of deep waters.
He rescued me from my powerful enemy,
from my foes, who were too
strong for me.
—Psalm 18:4–6, 16–17

Chemotherapy and death were my foes that were too strong for me, but God promised he would rescue me, and my terror subsided. As I continued to read his Word, the Psalms were echoing the cries of my heart to God:

I cry to you, O Lord;
I say, "You are my refuge," . . .
Listen to my cry,
for I am in desperate need;
rescue me from those who pursue me,

> *for they are too strong for me.*
> *Set me free from my prison,*
> *that I may praise your name.*
> —Psalm 142:5–7

Death and chemo were pursuing me, and they were much too strong for me alone. And the hospital bed was my prison.

> *O Lord, hear my prayer,*
> *listen to my cry for mercy;*
> *in your faithfulness and*
> *righteousness*
> *come to my relief. . . .*
> *I spread out my hands to you;*
> *my soul thirsts for you like a*
> *parched land.*
> *Answer me quickly, O Lord;*
> *my spirit fails. . . .*
> *Show me the way I should go,*
> *for to you I lift up my soul.*
> *Rescue me from my enemies,*
> *O Lord,*
> *for I hide myself in you. . . .*
> *For your name's sake, O Lord,*
> *preserve my life.*
> —Psalm 143:1, 6–9, 11

In that moment, my fear was gone and was replaced instead by a wonderful sense of absolute peace. I knew with a complete, unshakable assurance that my Lord would rescue me.

I didn't know *how,* only that he would.

Whether that meant healing me or taking me home to be with him, I was no longer afraid. For I belonged to the Lord.

I am his and nothing can change that.

Not cancer.

Not chemo.

Not death.

Yes, death could claim my cancer-ravaged and chemo-riddled body, but it could never touch my cancer-free soul.

The Lord promised that he would never leave me or forsake me, and he never has.

And I know that he never will. For that, I'm eternally grateful.

"For I know the plans I have for you," declares the LORD, "plans to prosper you and not to harm you, plans to give you hope and a future."
—JEREMIAH 29:11

thirteen

Laughter Is the Best Medicine

I'm living proof. Scientific studies show that laughter helps the healing process.

Humor is an affirmation of dignity, a declaration of man's superiority to all that befalls him.

—Romain Gary

In his 1979 pioneering book *Anatomy of an Illness* (W. W. Norton and Company, Inc., New York) Norman Cousins asserted that "laughter therapy" cured him from a crippling and supposedly irreversible disease. "Nothing is less funny than being flat on your back with all the bones in your spine and joints hurting," he wrote. But to check out his humor hypothesis, he began watching old Marx Brothers films and some of TV's *Candid Camera* classics while still in the hospital.

He discovered that ten minutes of genuine belly laughter had an anesthetic effect and would give him at least two hours of pain-free sleep.

More and more scientific studies in the past few decades have shown that humor increases alertness, stimulates the immune system, and even reduces pain. Today, countless doctors, nurses, and psychiatrists give seminars and presentations on the therapeutic benefits of humor.

The Bible *says* a cheerful heart is a good medicine (Prov. 17:22).

Well, I'm no doctor, medical scholar, or learned philosopher, but I'm a firm believer in the medicinal power of laughter.

I saw this firsthand the day I invited a small group of women over to my home for a little breast cancer survivor group tea party. As I was serving the tea (English-style with milk and sugar) I asked one of my guests, "One lump or two?"

"You don't ask that of a woman who's had breast cancer," said Sherris.

Every woman in the room—all who'd battled breast cancer—cracked up.

And the funny stories really started flowing with the tea.

Sherris, who had both chemo and radiation—which required x's marked on her upper chest and neck area in blue ink so the radiologist would know the right place to zap her with radiation—said that the kids in her son's kindergarten class would say to her: "Why do you have ink on you? You're not supposed to put ink on you!"

Then Lee shared the story of a friend's mother who had a mastectomy many years ago.

This active seventy-something mom lives in Hawaii and swims every day. The only problem is, her prosthesis keeps flipping out of her bathing suit.

"She's found it in all different pools—floating on top of the water," Lee said. "She just grabs it and stuffs it back in."

This vivid image set off more gales of laughter among the group. Especially when we all put our heads together to try to find a solution to the problem of the popping-out prosthesis.

"I wonder if Velcro would help?"

"Or a safety pin?"

"A button?"

"Maybe string?"

But Debbie came up with the best idea of all.

"She could write on it, 'If found, return to . . .' and put her name on it."

More peals of laughter.

A prosthesis isn't the only cancer accessory that doesn't behave quite the way we always want it to.

Debbie said she finally quit wearing a wig when a little girl in one of her classes said, "Teacher, why does your hair move when you turn your head?"

Janis can relate.

"I would scratch my head, and the wig would move back and forth. I'd be walking around asking people, 'Is my wig on straight?' I could never tell," she said.

Without her wig, Debbie recalled feeling like a character on *Star Trek*.

Although much of her hair had already fallen out, she still had some tufts remaining. In addition, she also had a catheter sticking out of one side of her chest and a plastic drain on the other side.

"I feel like one of the Borg," she told her husband. For those of you who aren't *Star Trek* fans, the Borg are creepy, pale, bald creatures—part-human, part-machine— with tubes sticking out of various parts of their bodies.

They walk around intoning, "We are Borg. You will be assimilated. Resistance is futile."

Unlike the Borg, Debbie does not believe that resistance is futile.

She fought back.

Then there was the woman who went in to see a brand-new doctor shortly after her mastectomy and reconstruction.

During the examination he looked in surprise at the large scar on her chest.

"Oh, that's not from my mastectomy; that's my appendectomy scar," she reassured him. Her plastic surgeon had performed what's known as a tram-flap procedure, the removal of a section of skin from her stomach; hence the appendectomy scar grafted onto her chest to form her new breast.

Joking with doctors and nurses is one of the *few* fun by-products of surgery.

Charlotte Frazier, seventy-four, said that during a recent chemo hospitalization, one of the nurses asked her if she'd like a sponge bath. "She brought me a washcloth to wash my face, and I said, 'Do you mind, I'd really like to wash and set my hair tonight,'" Charlotte recalled.

"The nurse looked at me and said, 'Huh?'

"I took the washcloth and wiped it over my bald head. Then I dried it and said, 'All through.'"

The nurse appreciated Charlotte's levity.

Lynda Duncan's known for her levity.

As her hair fell out from the chemo, she saved individual strands and taped them to index cards as a memento.

Lynda also got to the point during her many radiation and chemo treatments where she required that the hospital interns and residents meet her and make eye contact with her first before zeroing in on her chest.

And Bonnie Sheaffer joked with a doctor friend after having her mastectomy, "Well, I know that mammograms will hurt only half as much now."

It's nice when you can find a doctor with a sense of humor.

My aunt Annette had recuperated from her mastectomy and was fully dressed and waiting for her doctor to release her from the hospital. When he came in, he noticed her filled-out bra and asked her what she had stuffed it with.

"Kotex, cut in half," replied my ever-resourceful aunt.

"You never did know one end from the other," he laughed.

Laughter helps.

H'mmm, maybe that doctor was a colleague of Patch Adams.

The recent movie *Patch Adams* starring Robin Williams was based on the true story of a doctor who believed strongly in the healing power of humor and bucked the establishment of his time by doing goofy things to make his patients laugh.

147

One *Patch Adams* fan is sixty-year-old Barbara Nichols who went to see the movie with her friend Nancy on the advice of her doctor. The following week when Nancy took Barbara to her chemo treatment, the two women wore red plastic clown noses into the chemo room.

"Everyone started giggling, so I decided I'd just keep wearing the nose," Barbara said.

For the first time, people started looking forward to going to chemo.

Although I don't have a red plastic nose, if I'd been there I might have entertained the women with my little mammogram song. Please sing it with me again:

Thanks for the Mammogram

Thanks for the mammogram.
Though it hurt a little bit,
Okay, kind of a lot,
It's wonderful what it can do,
It found my cancer spot,
Now I'm cancer-free.
Thanks for the mammogram.
A small squish goes a long way
To finding the Big C.
It really can help save the life
Of folks like you and me.
Get your mam-mogram!

fourteen

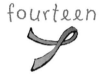

Where Do I Go from Here?

Helpful hints for women with breast cancer.

Nothing in life is to be feared. It is only to be understood.
—Madame Curie

By now you may be asking, "Where do I go from here?"

First, an important disclaimer that you've probably already figured out from reading this nonmedical book: I'm NOT a doctor, nurse, oncologist, or even a phlebotomist. In fact, I have to turn my head the other way when my blood is being drawn.

I did play *Operation!* as a kid if that counts though.

I'm simply an average, ordinary woman—just like you—who got breast cancer. And I well remember what it's like when you're first diagnosed; it can be a very frightening, overwhelming time. There's so much to learn; there are so many decisions to make and so many crazy emotions to deal with that you find yourself kind of fumbling through and learning as you go.

In an effort to cut through at least some of that confusion, I've created—with the help of some other breast cancer survivors—an informal list of helpful hints. It's by no means exhaustive (read the medical disclaimer above), and remember, I write humor, not deep, academic theses. This list highlights some of the important lessons we've learned that we wish someone had told us early on in our cancer journey.

151

1. First, find a doctor you trust—if you're not comfortable with your medical care, then change it. You need to believe in your doctor and feel that you're both on the same team aggressively fighting this disease together. Don't be afraid to ask questions.

2. Educate yourself about your breast cancer and the available treatments; ask for books or pamphlets from your doctor or local cancer organization. If you find all the information a bit overwhelming (and it *can* be), write down a list of questions and concerns to discuss with your doctor instead and take notes. Or have a friend take notes for you.

3. Learn to take charge of your treatment; don't let cancer be in control. Michael used to get frustrated with me because, in every other area of my life, I'm pretty assertive. But when it came to my cancer, I was initially passive, relinquishing all the control to the doctors and nurses since they were the "experts." However, as skilled as those in the medical profession may be, they are only human, and they can make mistakes. Remember, this is *your* body and *your* life we're talking about here.

4. Try to bring a friend or loved one along with you to all your doctor's appointments, chemo sessions, and

radiation treatments, both for emotional and purely practical reasons. Having two sets of ears to listen to what the doctor says helps, especially when you're in that chemo memory fog.

5. Seek out and talk to other women who have had breast cancer. If you don't know anyone who's had it, ask your doctor to refer you to someone, or check with your local chapter of the American Cancer Society.

6. Throw down your Wonder Woman cape and quit trying to do it all. Rest, take care of yourself, and let the noncritical things slide.

7. Don't be too proud to ask for help. Give your friends and family practical, specific tasks to do, such as cooking, laundry, and picking the kids up from school. Allow your loved ones this opportunity to show their love and support.

8. Talk openly to your loved ones about your cancer. Don't isolate yourself and think you have to be strong and hold things in. Be honest with them.

Additionally, there are many organizations available to provide answers to all of your cancer questions, a few of which I've listed below:

The American Cancer Society
800-ACS-2345 (800-227-2345)
Web site: www.cancer.org

National Alliance of Breast Cancer Organizations
(NABCO)
800-719-9154
Web site: www.nabco.org

National Cancer Institute
800-4-CANCER (800-422-6237)
Web site: cancernet.nci.nih.gov

The Susan G. Komen Breast Cancer Foundation
800-I'M-AWARE (800-462-9273)
Web site: www.breastcancerinfo.com

Y-Me National Breast Cancer Organization
twenty-four-hour hotline: 800-221-2141
Web site: www.y-me.org

There are also several breast cancer books on the market today, although I have to be honest and say I've deliberately *not* read them so I wouldn't be influenced in the writing of this book. But now that it's finished, I'm looking forward to checking some of them out, especially Rosie O'Donnell's *Bosom Buddies*. Therefore, I can't rate them for you. However, a search on amazon.com will give you both critical and readers' reviews.

Okay, okay, enough with the resource stuff; I almost felt like I was writing a term paper again. Time for me to get back on my "humor helps" soapbox.

Laughter works. Trust me.

Granted, humor's a very subjective thing. What I think is funny may not elicit even one giggle from you, and what others find hilarious may not even make me crack a smile. My former coworker Jeff absolutely loved The Three Stooges and Abbott and Costello, but they didn't do anything for me.

But, *I Love Lucy* gets me every time, as do reruns of the old *Dick Van Dyke Show*.

So what is it that makes *you* laugh?

Laurel and Hardy? *America's Funniest Home Videos*? Adam Sandler?

Maybe you're not a movie or TV person, so you get your laughs from the comic strips, say *Peanuts* or *Garfield*. Or maybe *The Far Side* (which Michael always had to explain to me until we got our dog, Gracie.)

Perhaps you enjoy just being around kids and seeing the funny things they do and say.

Pets can have the same effect. Gracie's always good for a few guffaws. Now I wish we'd had her when I was going through chemo; she's good for snuggling too.

And then there's the grande dame of humor: Erma Bombeck. I don't think I've ever met anyone who didn't enjoy Erma. She was the humor queen.

The important thing is to find the things that make you laugh and bring you joy and make them a part of your cancer experience.

Joy uplifts.

Joy seems to me a step beyond happiness—happiness is a sort of atmosphere you can live in sometimes when you're lucky. Joy is a light that fills you with hope and faith and love.

—Adela Rogers St. Johns

fifteen

Moms, Mammograms, and Other Things for Which I'm Thankful

A list of gratitude.

In gratitude for your own good fortune you must render in return some sacrifice of your life for other life.

—ALBERT SCHWEITZER

Going through cancer changes you. You start to think about what's really important. What really matters. And what you're thankful for. At least I did.

During one of my hospital stays I began making a list of thanks.

Here's the beginning of my list; I keep adding to it.

my breast cancer survivor mom

best friends named Lana

a husband who kissed my mastectomy scar when he saw it for the first time

Tostitos corn chips and Trader Joe's mild salsa

Dove ice-cream bars (milk chocolate, no nuts)

pantyhose that fit

Gene Kelly joyously splashing through puddles in *Singin' in the Rain*

afternoon naps

the Book of Psalms

that fresh baby-and-talcum-powder smell

long walks in the spring rain

compassionate nurses

pretending to be Barbra Streisand in *Funny Girl*
singing "Don't Rain on my Parade" at the top of
my lungs at 3 A.M. on the ferry from England to
France

no more peas!

plastic surgeons who do tattoos

having the breasts—or breast—of a twenty-two-year-
old again

a designer nipple made just for me

laughter

antinausea medication

health insurance

being able to stretch my arms wide enough to hug
my husband again

tap dancing

childlike wonder

warm chocolate pudding with the "skin" on top

imagination

someone to scratch the itch in that hard-to-reach
spot

skiing (okay, snowplowing) in the Swiss Alps

a gondola ride in Venice

that first breathless visit to the Louvre

seeing Yul Brynner in *The King and I* onstage in London's West End

neighborhood barbershops

that *Alien 3* came out *before* I went through chemo—thanks, Sigourney

friends and family who made or gave me pretty hats and scarves

the magic of makeup

Bob's Big Boy hamburgers

McDonald's French fries and chocolate shakes

Sunday afternoon drives in the country

kaleidoscopes

tilting at windmills and dreaming impossible dreams

a father who taught me to dream

a mother who encouraged those dreams

show-and-tell

Shirley Temple movies

dried roses, old photographs, dusty trunks from the attic, bits of lace, strands of pearls . . .

Mel Gibson in a kilt

a husband who told me I was beautiful when I was bald

California poppies

Double Delight roses and blue hydrangeas

suppositories (no, really!)

velour turbans to wear to bed at night to keep my head warm

the prayer of Saint Francis of Assisi

Wordsworth's ". . . hosts of golden daffodils . . ."

the man who loves the "pilgrim soul" in me

evening walks with Michael and our dog, Gracie

movie star heroes: John Wayne, Gary Cooper, Gregory Peck . . .

real heroes: The apostle Paul, Albert Schweitzer, my dad

a normal white blood cell count

The Statue of Liberty and what she means

flying a glider over the English countryside

the view of Paris from the Eiffel Tower

the Arc de Triomphe illuminated at night

clam chowder in sourdough bowls from San Francisco's Pier 39

whale watching in Monterey

being able to walk without pain

paper clips, white out, and back-up disks

no more math!

being able to go Christmas shopping without having to stop and rest every few minutes the sound of the wind rustling through the trees

Jimmy Stewart, Cary Grant, and Katharine Hepburn

the "It Pays to Increase Your Word Power" page in *Reader's Digest*

leaving the shark exhibit at Marine World with all my digital extremities intact

first-grade teachers named Miss Vopelinsky

waking up after surgery

heated blankets from the night shift nurse

bookmobiles and blissful grade-school hours spent in the library

favorite childhood friends: *Little Women, The Bobbsey Twins, Five Little Peppers and How They Grew,* the Betsy, Tacy and Tib books, Trixie Belden mysteries

graduating from college—finally—in my thirties

a child's sweet, sticky kiss

my little brother Todd who sang for quarters

my sister Lisa and our childhood canopy bed

that same sister who came over and gave me shots after my chemo treatments

silence

stimulating conversation

e-mail, pen pals, and postcards from far-off places

toasting marshmallows for s'mores and singing *"Kumbayah"* at summer camp

that there was no room in the inn

seeing Ginger Rogers and the Rockettes at Radio City Music Hall

that hair grows back

my brother-in-law Jim's Chateaubriand

cracked crab dipped in butter

fasting

heads bent in prayer

the strength to pump my own gas again

the opportunity to see Sammy Davis Jr. perform *Mr. Bojangles* LIVE!

England "my England"

hot buttered scones with strawberry jam and clotted cream and a "cuppa" tea

wandering through Yorkshire—James Herriott country

a perfect sentence

Louisa May Alcott and Laura Ingalls Wilder

kindred spirits

friends down the street who let me bathe in their tub when we had plumbing problems warm flannel nightgowns instead of those skimpy hospital gowns

C. S. Lewis and *The Chronicles of Narnia*

"Amazing Grace" on the bagpipes

Chinese takeout

reading in the tub

my mom bringing me chicken noodle soup, saltines, and warm 7-up when I'm sick

seeing Glenda Jackson in *Antony and Cleopatra* in Stratford-on-Avon

The Acropolis at night in Athens

a husband who changed my IV bag in the middle of the night

seeing *The Sound of Music* for the first time as a little girl in a big Chicago theater, especially the opening scene when Julie sings "The hills are alive . . ."

blissful Saturday afternoons at the National Gallery in London

Irish lilts, Scottish brogues, and *any* English accent

my grandma's sugary boiled frosting that cracked when you bit into it

that the vow "in sickness and in health" really means something

Girl Scout peanut butter patties—or Samoa's

sisters—and brothers-in-law—who helped in practical ways while I was recuperating

a prosthesis to give me that even-bosomed look again

squealing with excitement while trying to outrun the incoming tide

sixth-grade teachers named Miss Vanderbrug

my folks introducing me to Mario Lanza and MGM musicals when I was little

childhood field trips—The Chicago Museum of Science and Industry, that fifth-grade trip to the symphony

Handel's *Messiah*

string quartets playing Pachelbel's *Canon*

Linus reciting the Gospel of Luke in *A Charlie Brown Christmas*

"Now I lay me down to sleep . . ."

answered prayer

seeing the Boston Pops LIVE on the Fourth of July—on Boston Common

nobody but Judy singing "Over the Rainbow"

Mandy Patinkin singing "Lily's Eyes" from *The Secret Garden*

not being hooked up to an IV any longer

camping at Calaveras Big Trees with Michael

visiting fifteen countries before I was twenty-three
   years old

swimming in the deep turquoise of the Mediter-
   ranean

the pigeons scattering at St. Mark's Square in Venice

seeing Van Gogh's "starry, starry night"

so many Rembrandts at the Rijksmuseum
   in Amsterdam

the train ride from Oxford to London

Beethoven's Ninth Symphony

Patsy Cline singing "Crazy"

a great metaphor

that the tomb was empty

being able to roll over and sleep on my side again

kringle (fabulous Danish pastry) from my hometown
   of Racine, Wisconsin

Anne Frank's diary

books that stay with you long after you've put them
   down

a child's hand nestled trustingly in mine

waiting 'til the wedding night

a love that grows deeper over time

"whither thou goest, I will go . . ."

Mother Teresa

Corrie ten Boom and *The Hiding Place*

kind, skilled surgeons

doctors with great bedside manners

the days when carhops brought mugs of frosted root
  beer to your car

Debbie Reynolds singing "Tammy's in Love"

seeing *The Little Mermaid* in Copenhagen harbor

Junior Mints, buttered popcorn, and a cherry Coke
  at the movies

seeing Rosemary Clooney LIVE!

regaining my stamina for fun Trivial Pursuit nights
  with friends

seeing the Northern Lights from the cockpit
  of an Air Force C-141

watching the sun set over the ocean at Point Reyes
  with Michael

secondhand bookstores

George MacDonald's *Sir Gibbie*

My Utmost for His Highest

that first heart-stopping glimpse of the Venus de
  Milo

seeing Monet's water lilies up close and personal

a father who stepped to his "different drummer"

listening to my own "different drummer"

that Jesus wept

knowing I'll *never forget* after visiting Dachau

favorite aunts

women who generously showed me their
rebuilt breasts

strolling along the Seine

sunbathing on the Greek Isles

being mesmerized by the eight-hour theatrical
experience of *Nicholas Nickleby* at The Great
Lakes Shakespeare Festival in Cleveland, Ohio

my marriage to a fellow artist

eleven pink tulips and one red one

the power of dreams

that I was my father's *Yenta Mi* (Danish
for "my little girl")

no more final exams

the UPS truck stopping at the front door

midnight services on Christmas Eve

my "baby" brother Tim with the curly hair

the privilege of living in England for three years

Rachmaninoff's *Rhapsody on a Theme of Paganini*

that joyous rush of recognition upon seeing
Gainsborough's portrait of Sarah Siddons

in London after reading about it many years earlier
as a young girl in Wisconsin

The Girl of the Limberlost

Bobby Darin singing "Mack the Knife"

Billy Graham

receiving the news of my first book contract
just in time for my fortieth birthday

royalty checks

another year cancer-free

For information about speaking engagements, retreats, luncheons, or one-day events, please contact Laura Jensen Walker c/o Revell Publicity (or e-mail Laura at Ljenwalk@aol.com).